Orthopaedic Emergencies

John T. Gorczyca

Orthopaedic Emergencies

A Manual for Medical Students, Physicians, PAs and NPs

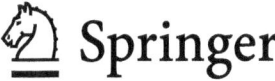 Springer

John T. Gorczyca
Department of Orthopedics
University of Rochester Medical Center
Rochester, NY, USA

ISBN 978-3-031-62010-2   ISBN 978-3-031-62011-9   (eBook)
https://doi.org/10.1007/978-3-031-62011-9

© The Editor(s) (if applicable) and The Author(s), under exclusive license to
Springer Nature Switzerland AG 2024
This work is subject to copyright. All rights are solely and exclusively licensed by
the Publisher, whether the whole or part of the material is concerned, specifically
the rights of translation, reprinting, reuse of illustrations, recitation, broadcasting,
reproduction on microfilms or in any other physical way, and transmission or
information storage and retrieval, electronic adaptation, computer software, or by
similar or dissimilar methodology now known or hereafter developed.
The use of general descriptive names, registered names, trademarks, service
marks, etc. in this publication does not imply, even in the absence of a specific
statement, that such names are exempt from the relevant protective laws and
regulations and therefore free for general use.
The publisher, the authors and the editors are safe to assume that the advice and
information in this book are believed to be true and accurate at the date of
publication. Neither the publisher nor the authors or the editors give a warranty,
expressed or implied, with respect to the material contained herein or for any
errors or omissions that may have been made. The publisher remains neutral with
regard to jurisdictional claims in published maps and institutional affiliations.

This Springer imprint is published by the registered company Springer Nature
Switzerland AG
The registered company address is: Gewerbestrasse 11, 6330 Cham, Switzerland

If disposing of this product, please recycle the paper.

Contents

Unstable Pelvic Fracture

1

A 25-year-old male is involved in a motorcycle cycle accident in which he strikes a utility pole. He arrives in the emergency department awake and alert with a HR of 108 bpm and blood pressure 80/52 mmHg. He complains of pain in his pelvic area. His initial anteroposterior (AP) X-ray of the pelvis is shown (Fig. 1.1). What is his likelihood that he will die from this injury?

This patient is hemodynamically unstable and has an unstable pelvis fracture. His expected mortality rate is 25% [1]. This is a fairly high mortality rate for a traumatic injury.

Why is the mortality rate so high?

Pelvis injuries tend to bleed, and displaced (mechanically unstable) pelvis injuries bleed more. The bleeding comes from the fracture, from the traumatized venous plexus anterior to the sacral bone at the posterior pelvis, and occasionally from injury to the arteries of the pelvis [2]. Total blood loss from an unstable pelvis fracture can be as high as 4–6 units (2–3 l) of blood, which can result in death by exsanguination [1]. Typically, blood volume is 7% of a patient's mass, so a 70 kg patient will have a blood volume of 4.9 l, and could lose more than half of that from the unstable pelvis injury alone.

Additionally, patients with pelvic fractures often have other injuries that contribute to the high mortality rate.

© The Author(s), under exclusive license to Springer Nature
Switzerland AG 2024
J. T. Gorczyca, *Orthopaedic Emergencies*,
https://doi.org/10.1007/978-3-031-62011-9_1

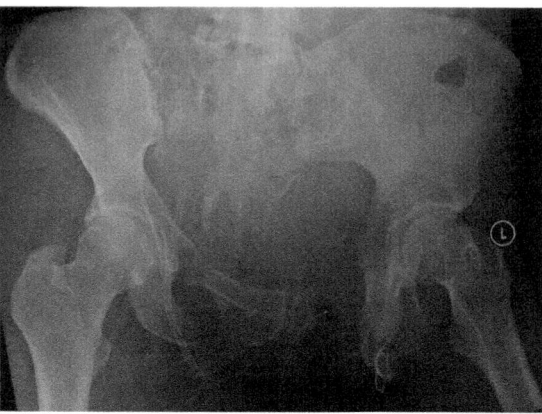

Fig. 1.1 Anteroposterior (AP) radiograph of the pelvis demonstrates obvious diastasis at the anterior pelvis, with more subtle findings of left sacral fracture and right sacroiliac joint displacement. This amount of displacement (>2.5 cm anteriorly and >1 cm posteriorly) is indicative of an unstable pelvis injury that has a high capacity for hemorrhage, warrants close hemodynamic monitoring and aggressive resuscitation as needed, benefits from provisional external stabilization of the pelvis, and ultimately is treated with definitive surgical stabilization when the patient is stable enough to have surgery

What are the radiographic features that mark this pelvis injury as having the potential to bleed significantly?

In general, pelvis injuries that have displacement of the posterior pelvis (in the sacroiliac region) on the initial AP pelvis X-ray have sustained enough force to cause not only displacement of the fracture, but also disruption of the soft tissues and vascular plexus anterior to the sacroiliac region [2, 3] (Fig. 1.2). Thus, displacement of the posterior pelvis by 1 cm or more on the initial AP pelvis X-ray taken in the trauma bay will identify patients at risk for significant hemorrhage and serves as an important piece of information in the prioritization of this patient's care.

Fractures with more than 2.5 cm separation (diastasis) of the anterior pelvis at the pubic symphysis are also at risk for significant hemorrhage [4]. It has been demonstrated in the laboratory that in order for a pubic symphyseal diastasis of 2.5 cm to occur,

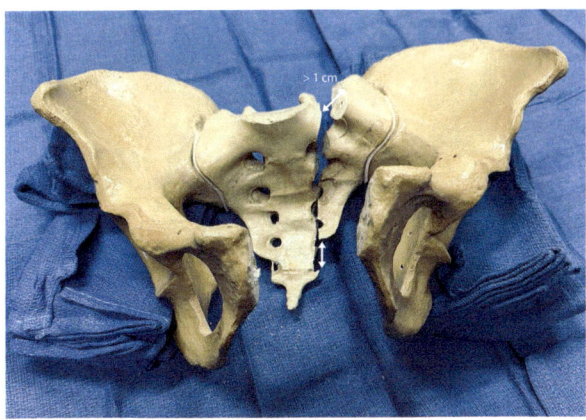

Fig. 1.2 Sawbone pelvis model depicts pelvis fracture with displacement at pubic symphysis anteriorly as well as at the left sacrum posteriorly. The displacement of the fracture >1 cm posteriorly is disruptive to the stabilizing soft tissues, numerous blood vessels, and in some cases, the nerves in the vicinity

there must be disruption of at least the anterior sacroiliac ligaments at the posterior pelvis, which in turn is associated with disruption of the posterior pelvis venous plexus and significant hemorrhage. Thus, this "open book pelvis" injury in this patient is associated with significant hemorrhage (Fig. 1.3).

Initial radiographs can be misleading because some severe pelvis injuries with significant displacement at the time of impact will recoil or will assume an alignment that is less displaced at the time that the X-ray is taken. In some cases, the instability of the pelvis can be detected by physical examination or by CT scan. It is prudent to assume that a pelvis injury is mechanically unstable in the early evaluation and resuscitation of trauma patients. It is for this reason that many EMTs and paramedics will presumptively place an external pelvis immobilizer on a patient based on the nature of the accident (e.g., fall greater than 10 feet, motor vehicle collision with greater than one foot of intrusion, MVC in which the patient is ejected from the vehicle, and motorcycle accident).

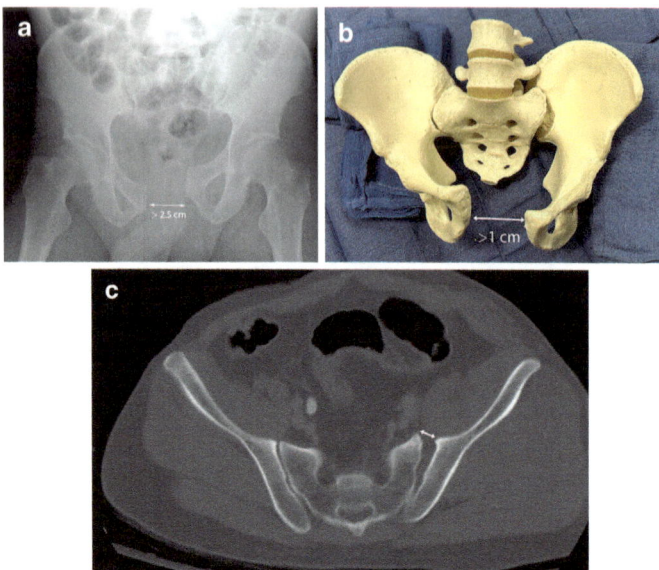

Fig. 1.3 (**a**) AP pelvis radiograph demonstrates classic "open book pelvis fracture" with diastasis (separation) of the pubic symphysis >2.5 cm, which is pathognomonic for pelvic instability and potential for significant hemorrhage. (**b**) Bone model depicts pubic symphysis diastasis and anterior sacroiliac joint displacement. Although the posterior sacroiliac ligaments are not disrupted in this case, the displacement at the anterior aspect of the sacroiliac joint is associated with mechanical instability and significant hemorrhage. (**c**) CT scan demonstrates sacroiliac joint in open book pelvis injury, with displacement anteriorly despite intact posterior ligaments, which function like the binding of a book when the book is opened

For a pelvis fracture with an unclear degree of instability after X-rays, physical examination, and CT scan, stress evaluation of the pelvis with fluoroscopy can be helpful in identifying which of the patients with a minimally displaced injury on initial x-ray have an unstable injury that has the ongoing potential for significant hemorrhage, and determining whether or not surgery should be performed to stabilize the pelvis (Fig. 1.4).

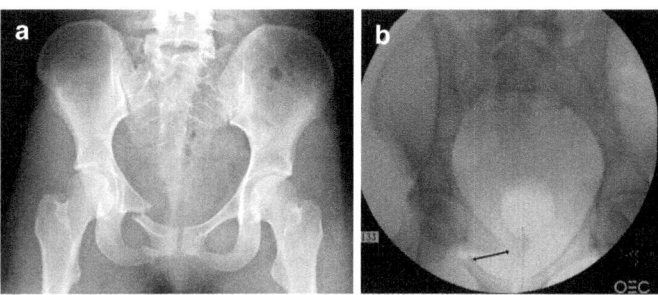

Fig. 1.4 (**a**) AP pelvis radiograph has displacement at right superior pubic ramus fracture. The exact degree of instability is unclear. (**b**) Intraoperative "stress" radiographs show significantly more displacement at the superior pubic ramus (black arrow) and establish that there is significant instability of the fracture

What steps should be taken to maximize survival of this patient?

After assuring that the patient has an adequate airway and is breathing and ventilating well, the next priority is his circulation. The patient should be treated with immediate resuscitation using intravenous fluids and/or blood products and by provisionally stabilizing the pelvis [1].

The first step in this resuscitation involves obtaining intravenous access and administering fluids.

Provisional stabilization of the pelvis can be provided by tightly wrapping a sheet around the pelvis or by a using a circumferential pelvic band which, when tightened will, decrease the size of the pelvic ring, and provide enough stability to the pelvic tissues to facilitate stable clot formation (Fig. 1.5). The net effect will be to decrease the rate of hemorrhage as much as possible so that the patient can respond to the intravenous fluids and blood products.

What fluids should this patient receive for resuscitation?

This patient has a systolic BP <90 mmHg and a HR >100 bpm, either of which by itself meets the criteria for hemodynamic instability and according to ATLS guidelines, and warrants an immedi-

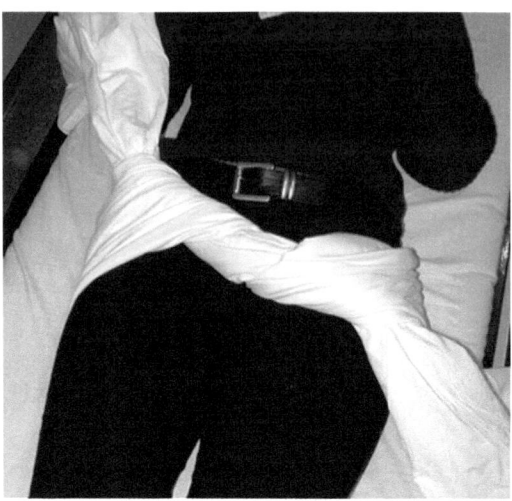

Fig. 1.5 Photograph depicts the position of a simple sheet that is wrapped and tightened around the pelvis in a model patient in order to provide some stability to the pelvis. Note that in an actual patient, the clothing would have been removed

ate bolus of 1000 cc crystalloid solution (lactated Ringers solution or 1/2 normal saline). This serves as a quick means to improve the patient's intravascular volume and evaluates the degree of hemodynamic instability to determine the need for further resuscitation. If the patient's vital signs improve enough that they become hemodynamically stable and remain hemodynamically stable, then the bolus was effective. If the patient becomes hemodynamically stable and later drifts into hemodynamic instability, then further resuscitation will be necessary. The worst possibility is if the patient's hemodynamic status does not return to the normal range after the initial bolus—in this case, the patient is in critical danger and immediate further resuscitation with packed red blood cells (PRBCs) and other blood products is essential. Early identification of the patient who will not respond to the initial bolus is crucial to their survival, and it is for this reason that the entire initial liter of intravenous fluid should be infused as quickly as possible—the patient's life will depend on it [5].

Figure 1.6 depicts a patient with an unstable pelvis injury while in the ICU the day following injury. What else do you see that will affect this patient's survival rate?

In addition to the pelvic binder, the patient has (1) a chest tube indicative of hemothorax and or pneumothorax. This is typically caused by rib fractures caused by significant force to the chest wall, which usually causes pulmonary contusion and explains the (2) endotracheal tube and mechanical ventilation. He also has a (3) sterile seal/dressing covering his open abdomen which could not be closed after emergency laparotomy due to post-ischemic swelling of the abdominal organs which would cause elevated intra-abdominal pressure and impaired organ perfusion (i.e., abdominal compartment syndrome). (4) A cervical collar is in place as a cervical spine injury has not yet been ruled out. This polytrauma patient with an unstable pelvis is not unusual in the number of associated injuries, and it is the constellation of injuries in such patients that contributes to the high mortality rate.

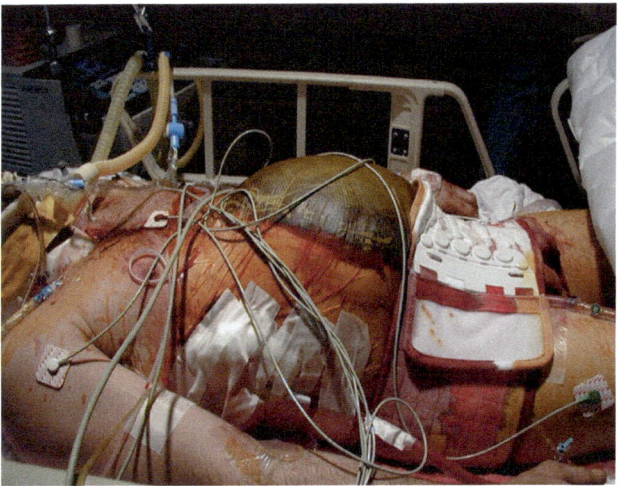

Fig. 1.6 Photograph of trauma patient with unstable pelvis fracture in pelvic immobilizing device the day following injury. Note that the patient appears to have multiple other injuries, which is not unusual when patients have pelvic fractures, and contributes to the high mortality rate of patients with unstable pelvis fractures

Figure 1.7 shows an unstable pelvis injury and a common iliac artery occlusion. The artery was repaired and circulation was returned to the leg. How long will this patient be at risk of significant hemorrhage?

The risk of hemorrhage is high at the time of injury, at the time of resuscitation, and remains high until after the unstable injury is operatively stabilized. This particular patient remained critically unstable for 5 days after injury, and on the sixth day, during open reduction of the pelvis, died from exsanguination. Thus, the risk of significant hemorrhage can last many days, and patients are at risk of exsanguination at the scene of the accident, in the Emergency Room resuscitation bay, in the Intensive Care unit, and in the operating room.

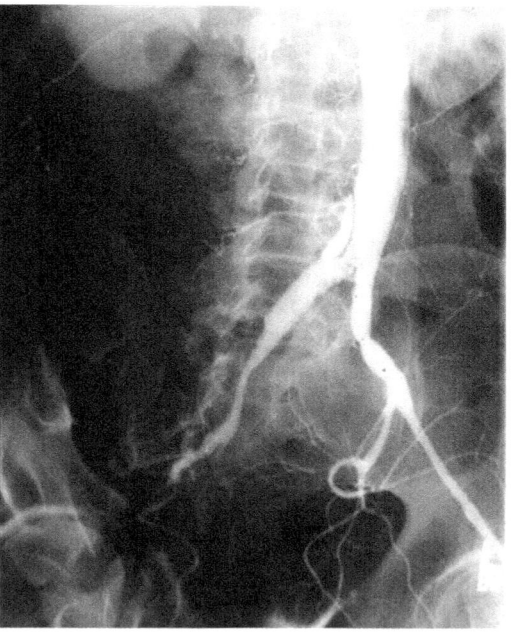

Fig. 1.7 AP lumbosacral spine radiograph depicts markedly unstable right iliac fracture and thrombosed external and internal iliac arteries. This patient ultimately exsanguinated from the pelvis fracture

Figure 1.8 shows the radiograph of a patient with an unstable, complex pelvis fracture with a pubic symphysis diastasis. What are some of the benefits of surgery for this patient?

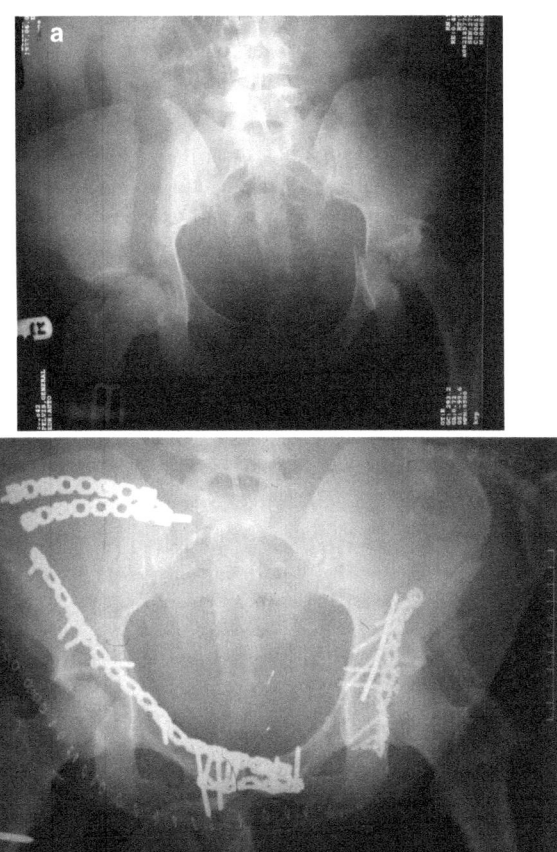

Fig. 1.8 (**a**) AP pelvis radiograph demonstrates highly unstable bilateral pelvis injury. Surgery is warranted to stabilize the pelvis to decrease ongoing hemorrhage, to improve comfort, and to restore alignment of the pelvis. (**b**) AP pelvis radiograph taken postoperatively demonstrates the extent of the stabilization procedure that was required for this pelvis injury

(1) Surgery to stabilize the mechanically unstable pelvis will control motion of the pelvis and thus decrease the risk of ongoing hemorrhage; (2) decrease the amount of pain experienced when the patient moves, allowing repositioning for improved pulmonary and skin care; (3) restore alignment of the pelvis for proper healing, which is associated with improved long term functional outcomes.

How does the shape of the pelvis affect its mechanics and surgical considerations?

The pelvis is a bony-ligamentous ring comprised of the sacrum and the two innominate bones, which are connected to each other by the pubic symphysis anteriorly and to each side of the sacrum posteriorly by the sacroiliac ligamentous complex. When the ligaments are disrupted or the bone is fractured and displaced, the displaced area should be realigned ("reduced") and held in place with plates and screws (or in some cases by an external fixation system, although these are being used less frequently these days). The plates and screws are not strong enough to allow the patient to stand or walk on the side(s) of the injury, so the patient will be mobilized with restricted weight bearing on one or both lower extremities for 2–3 months until the fracture has healed (Fig. 1.9). Once the injury has healed, it may take 2 more months for the patient to regain enough strength, comfort, and balance control to walk without any assistive devices (Fig. 1.10).

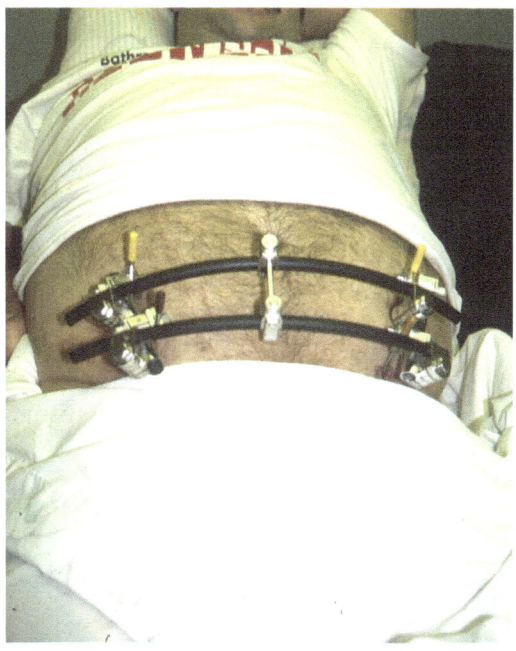

Fig. 1.9 Clinical photograph demonstrates external fixator that was on this patient who was non-weight bearing until the fracture healed in 3 months

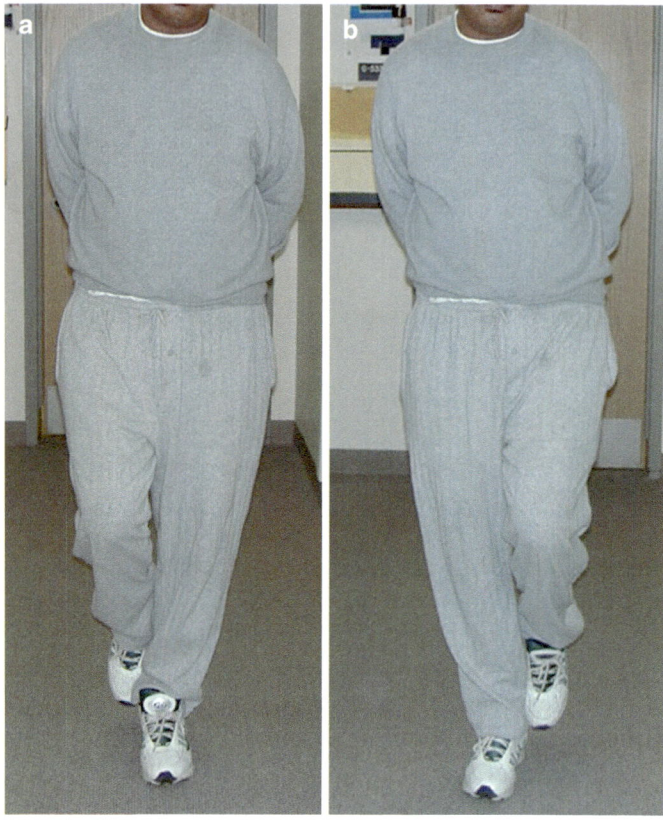

Fig. 1.10 Clinical photographs of patient 5 months after surgery bearing full weight on each leg individually (**a, b**). He initially was restricted from bearing weight for 3 months until the fracture healed, and it took another 2 months before he could bear full weight in a single-leg stance, which is necessary in order to walk without assistance

References

1. American College of Surgeons Committee on Trauma. Advanced trauma life support: student course manual. 10th ed. Chicago: American College of Surgeons; 2018.
2. Tile M. Pelvic ring fractures: should they be fixed? J Bone Joint Surg Br. 1988;70(1):1–12. https://doi.org/10.1302/0301-620X.70B1.3276697.
3. Langford JR, Burgess AR, Liporace FA, Haidukewych GJ. Pelvic fractures: part 1. Evaluation, classification, and resuscitation. J Am Acad Orthop Surg. 2013;21(8):448–57. https://doi.org/10.5435/JAAOS-21-08-448.
4. Young JW, Burgess AR, Brumback RJ, Poka A. Pelvic fractures: value of plain radiography in early assessment and management. Radiology. 1986;160(2):445–51. https://doi.org/10.1148/radiology.160.2.3726125.
5. Hak DJ, Smith WR, Suzuki T. Management of hemorrhage in life-threatening pelvic fracture. J Am Acad Orthop Surg. 2009;17(7):447–57. https://doi.org/10.5435/00124635-200907000-00005.

Traumatic Amputation

A man is run over by a train and sustains bilateral amputa-tions (Fig. 2.1). What would be the most likely cause of death from this injury?

Traumatic amputation is associated with massive hemorrhage and death from exsanguination [1, 2]. Other potential problems are infection from the open wound, and loss of function due to the loss of the amputated limb [3].

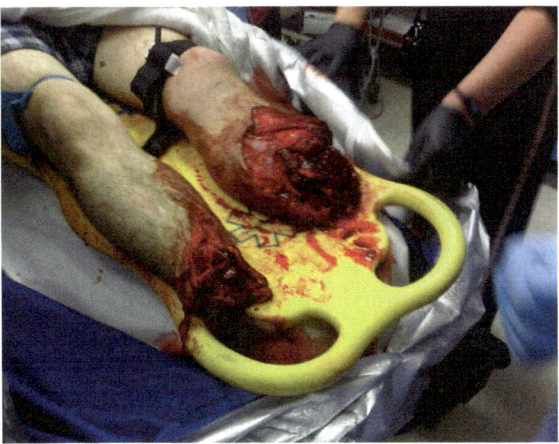

Fig. 2.1 Clinical photograph demonstrates traumatic below knee amputation, which is at high risk for severe hemorrhage and requires some form of pressure to control the bleeding. In this patient, a tourniquet has been applied to the thigh

© The Author(s), under exclusive license to Springer Nature Switzerland AG 2024

J. T. Gorczyca, *Orthopaedic Emergencies*,

https://doi.org/10.1007/978-3-031-62011-9_2

What can be done to control bleeding?

It is essential that bleeding is controlled early and effectively in order to maximize chances for survival. In many cases, direct pressure over the wound or compression of the main artery proximal to a wound (proximal arterial pressure) will control hemorrhage. Applying and inflating/tightening a tourniquet to the amputated limb(s) can achieve effective control of hemorrhage, and if it is secured in the tightened position, will not require a person to continue to apply pressure.

Rapid application of tourniquets can be lifesaving, especially with devastating injuries from explosives, high-energy gunshot wounds, and cases of multiple extremity wounds.

Tourniquets work by applying a tight circumferential force around the extremity to squeeze and compress the vessels. Unfortunately, the tourniquet, if left in place for a long time, can cause necrosis of all tissue distal to the level of the tourniquet. Extensive necrosis of skin and soft tissue caused by prolonged use of a tourniquet may necessitate a higher level of amputation and consequent functional loss. Thus, tourniquets should not be used for longer than is necessary. The sooner the tourniquet can safely be removed, the better the chances for optimal function of the residual (amputated) limb [4].

Occasionally, an amputated body part can be successfully reattached (replanted) after amputation.

What should be done to preserve the amputated body part in order to assure the greatest chance of successful replantation?

The amputated body part should be quickly cleaned of gross debris, protected from drying by wrapping it in a moistened gauze or clean towel, and placed in a clear plastic bag for easy identification. In order to preserve the viability of the tissue, the body part should be cooled as much as possible by placing it in a clear plastic bag on crushed ice or in ice water. The body part should be transported to the medical center as quickly as possible, with the patient whenever possible.

The above thru-forearm amputation was delivered to the hospital with the patient in hopes of replantation to restore

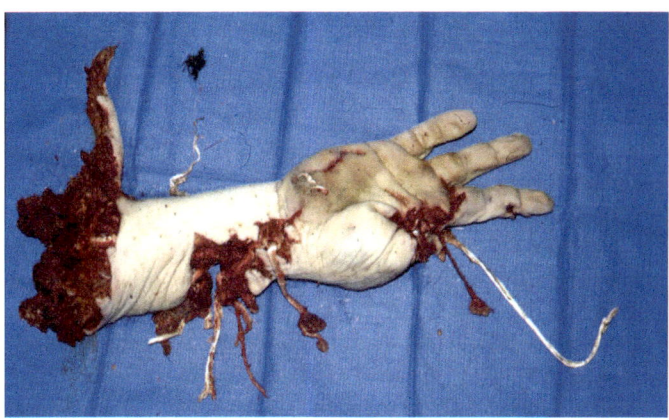

Fig. 2.2 Clinical photograph of a forearm amputation in a 58-year-old man sustained in a sawmill accident. The injury occurs in two areas of the forearm (i.e., segmental), there is tissue loss, muscle is crushed, the thumb and index finger are missing, the tendons are torn, and all neurovascular structures have been transected in at least one area. This is unlikely to have a good result if replantation is attempted

function (Fig. 2.2). What factors make this amputated limb unlikely to undergo successful replantation?

This limb has multiple irregular wounds with evidence of crushing. In addition to the forearm amputation, two of the fingers are amputated. There is gross contamination. Multiple nerves and vessels are transected. The tendons are traumatized. Clean cut amputations at a single level are more likely to undergo successful replantation. The more distal in the extremity the amputation occurs, the greater the chance for successful replantation [5].

What are the best indications for replantation of an amputated body part?

Children are more likely than adults to successfully heal replanted body parts, regenerate nerves and vessels, and achieve beneficial function after replantation. Thus, it is desirable to attempt replantation of almost any amputated body part in children. Older patients with medical comorbidities such as diabetes and vascular disease are less likely to have successful replantation surgery and have a shorter lifespan in which to experience any benefit, so replantation is less likely to be the appropriate treatment option.

The most important of the five fingers is the thumb, as it functions to oppose the other fingers when an object is gripped. Even when the thumb has minimal motion and sensation, it serves an important function, so almost every thumb amputation should be replanted. Amputation of any of the other digits can be tolerated as most people can function well with three fingers and a thumb. Amputation of multiple fingers, however, is a good indication for replantation of one or more digits.

When a decision is made not to replant an amputated body part (Fig. 2.3), what should be done at the time of surgery?

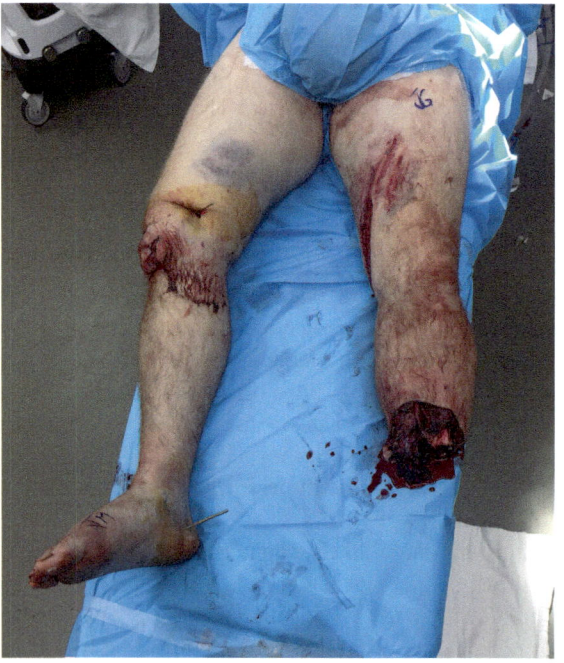

Fig. 2.3 Intraoperative photograph of traumatic amputation that requires debridement of devitalized bone and wound closure. Sometimes, it is necessary to shorten the bone to allow tissue closure

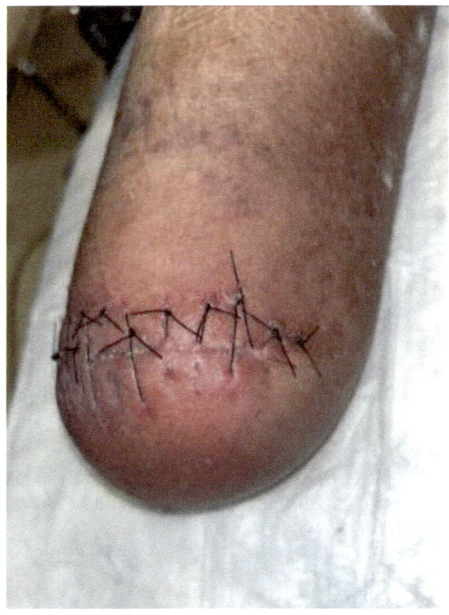

Fig. 2.4 Clinical photograph of residual limb 6 weeks after below knee amputation. The skin is now healed enough to allow removal of the sutures

Surgery after amputation is performed to remove devitalized tissue, irrigate the contaminated tissue, ligate the transected blood vessels, allow the nerves to retract so they do not get entrapped in scar and create a painful neuroma, shorten the bone to the appropriate level for healing and function, and cover the bone with soft tissue and skin to make a durable sensate surface for weight bearing and prosthetic wear (Fig. 2.4). Sutures should be left in place for 4–6 weeks after amputation to assure proper healing of the tissue before fitting the patient for a prosthesis.

References

1. DellaVope J, Simms E, Heaney JB, Guice J, McSwain N Jr, Meade P, Duchesne JC. Impact of inverse ratios on patients with exsanguinating vascular injuries: should more be the new paradigm? J Trauma Acute Care Surg. 2013;74(2):403–9. https://doi.org/10.1097/TA.0b013e31827e210b.
2. Passos E, Dingley B, Smith A, Engels PT, Ball CG, Faidi S, Nathens A, Tien H, Canadian Trauma Trials Collaborative. Tourniquet use for peripheral vascular injuries in the civilian setting. Injury. 2014;45(3):573–7. https://doi.org/10.1016/j.injury.2013.11.031. Epub 2013 Dec 4.
3. Harris AM, Althausen PL, Kellam J, Bosse MJ, Castillo R, Lower Extremity Assessment Project (LEAP) Study Group. Complications following limb-threatening lower extremity trauma. J Orthop Trauma. 2009;23(1):1–6. https://doi.org/10.1097/BOT.0b013e31818e43dd.
4. Aucar JA, Hirshberg A. Damage control for vascular injuries. Surg Clin North Am. 1997;77(4):853–62. https://doi.org/10.1016/s0039-6109(05)70589-2.
5. Boulas HJ. Amputations of the fingers and hand: indications for replantation. J Am Acad Orthop Surg. 1998;6(2):100–5. https://doi.org/10.5435/00124635-199803000-00004.

Femoral Shaft Fractures

3

A 24-year-old male is involved in an ATV accident and sustains an isolated femur fracture. Initial chest X-ray shows no rib fractures, contusion, pneumothorax, or hemothorax. His initial femur radiograph is shown (Fig. 3.1). What are the mechanical characteristics of the femur and how will this affect the patient's evaluation and treatment?

The femur is the longest and strongest bone in the human body. It is tubular in shape, which makes it able to withstand significant forces of rotation, bending in any direction, and axial load. It is surrounded by some of the strongest muscles in the body (the quadriceps femoris anteriorly and the hamstring muscles posteriorly) which have an abundant blood supply. The central intramedullary canal contains marrow, the nutrient artery of the femur, and cancellous bone. The dense cortical bone on the outer periphery and the surrounding periosteum also has blood vessels that can bleed significantly after fracture.

Thus, it requires a significant force to fracture the femur, and that force will often result in associated injuries that may not be immediately apparent. Additionally, the highly vascular femur and its surrounding tissues can bleed significantly and cause hypotension, shock, and death. Patients with femoral shaft fractures should be evaluated as trauma patients according to protocols established by ATLS [1], and their resuscitation should likewise follow ATLS guidelines.

© The Author(s), under exclusive license to Springer Nature   21
Switzerland AG 2024
J. T. Gorczyca, *Orthopaedic Emergencies*,
https://doi.org/10.1007/978-3-031-62011-9_3

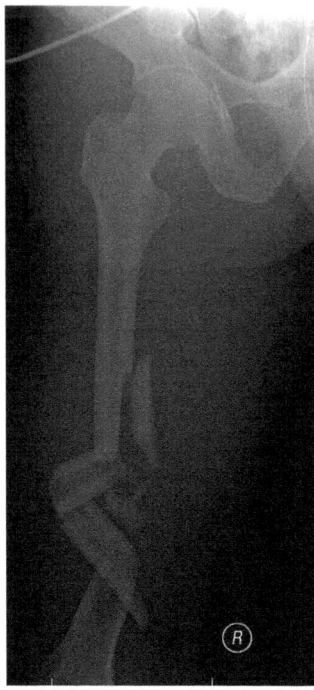

Fig. 3.1 Anteroposterior (AP) radiograph of the femoral shaft demonstrates multiple bony fragments (comminution). This radiograph also demonstrates a minimally displaced fracture at the base of the femoral neck. The femur is the longest and strongest bone in the body, and its tubular shape makes it able to withstand significant force. It takes a significant traumatic event to create a fracture like this in the femur, and there are likely to be associated injuries to other body parts, warranting thorough evaluation and re-examination of the patient. The patient is also at risk for significant hemorrhage (2–3 units) from the femur fracture

What is the risk of mortality in patients with femoral shaft fractures?

The mortality risk of patients with femoral shaft fractures is dependent on many factors, the most important being the other associated injuries. An isolated femur fracture has a fairly low mortality risk, but patients with bilateral femoral shaft fractures have a mortality risk of approximately 25%, which is in large part due to the associated injuries (e.g., brain, lung, chest wall, abdominal organs, pelvis) in these patients [1, 2]. Of note, the 25% mortality risk of bilateral femur fractures (each of which has the potential of 2–3 units blood loss) is the same as that of the unstable patient with an unstable pelvis fracture, which has a potential blood loss of 4–6 units of blood. The Injury Severity Score (ISS) is a system that is used to grade injuries in multiple organ systems and calculates a score which, when factoring in the patient's age, can be used to predict risk of mortality [1].

What should be done acutely to help the patient with a femoral fracture?

First, the patient undergoes the primary survey evaluation according to ATLS guidelines to assure that the airway and breathing are stable, and that obvious bleeding is controlled. The femur fracture is usually apparent on secondary survey due to the significant deformity, swelling, and discomfort present (Fig. 3.2). Next, the femoral shaft fracture should be reduced (realigned) and

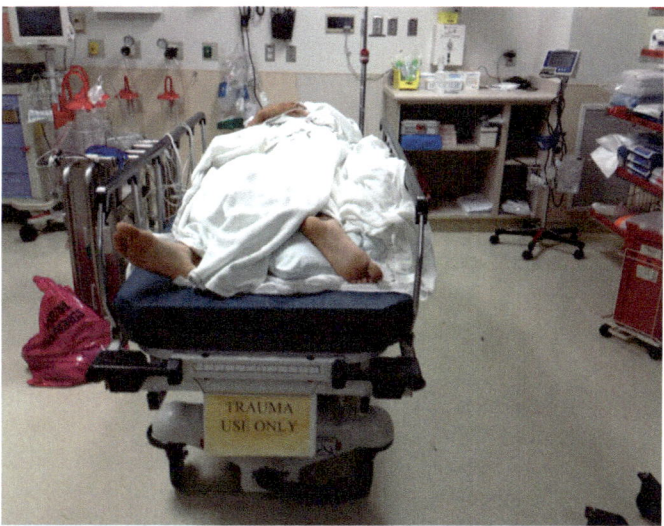

Fig. 3.2 Clinical photograph of a patient with femur fracture demonstrates significant rotational displacement and shortening of the left femur, clearly showing that a major injury has occurred to the extremity

held in that position. With most long bone fractures other than the femur, the extremity can be held in a reduced position by aligning the fracture and immobilizing the bone and the joint proximal and distal to it, often with some type of splint. But the femur is different because the large and powerful quadriceps and hamstring muscles in the region of the fracture contract in response to the injury and prevent maintenance of proper alignment and maintenance of position. Thus, the early treatment of the femoral shaft fracture is best performed by using traction, generally using a Hare traction splint initially (Fig. 3.3a), and occasionally skeletal traction, which is achieved with traction through a wire or pin which is placed through the femur or tibia distal to the fracture (Fig. 3.3b).

What are the benefits of traction in the early treatment of femoral shaft fracture?

Traction will achieve several important goals: It will decrease the size of the thigh compartment and will thus decrease the capacity for hemorrhage; it will stabilize the femur so that there is less motion, thereby decreasing ongoing hemorrhage and the risk of injury to muscle, skin and neurovascular structures by motion of the sharp bony fragments; it will make the patient more comfortable; it will in some cases improve distal circulation by straightening kinked or deformed blood vessels and restoring proper perfusion to the distal extremity; and it will facilitate later surgery by not allowing contracture of the tissues, thereby making it easier to attain the proper length of the femur intraoperatively.

Figure 3.4a, b demonstrate the femur and initial chest X-ray of an 18-year-old patient who sustained an isolated femur fracture in a motocross accident. Head, neck, chest, and abdominal/pelvic CT scans were negative. He was placed in skeletal traction and received analgesic medication. Operative stabilization of his femoral shaft fracture was postponed for various reasons on each of the following 3 days. On the fourth day, he demonstrated confusion in the preoperative area.

What is the likely cause of the patient's confusion?

There are multiple potential causes of confusion, but the most likely at that time point in a healthy young patient with unstabilized long bone fractures is hypoxia from fat embolism syndrome.

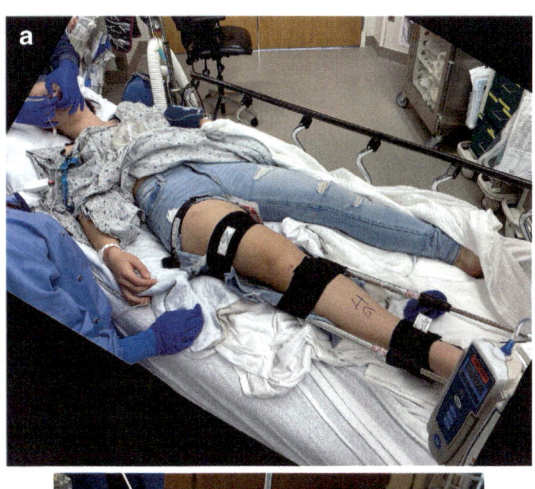

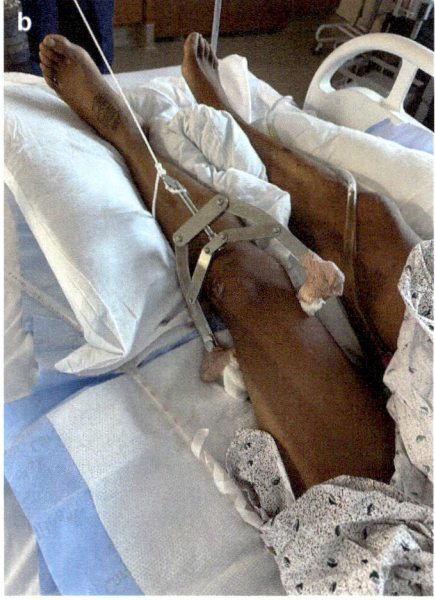

Fig. 3.3 (**a**) Hare traction splint that had been applied by emergency medical technicians (EMTs) at the scene of a motor vehicle accident in which the patient sustained an apparent femoral shaft fracture. The traction will improve comfort, decrease blood loss, prevent ongoing tissue injury, and make it easier to obtain proper reduction of the fracture at the time of surgery. (**b**) Traction pin placed in the distal femur in a patient allows traction to be applied to the extremity preoperatively

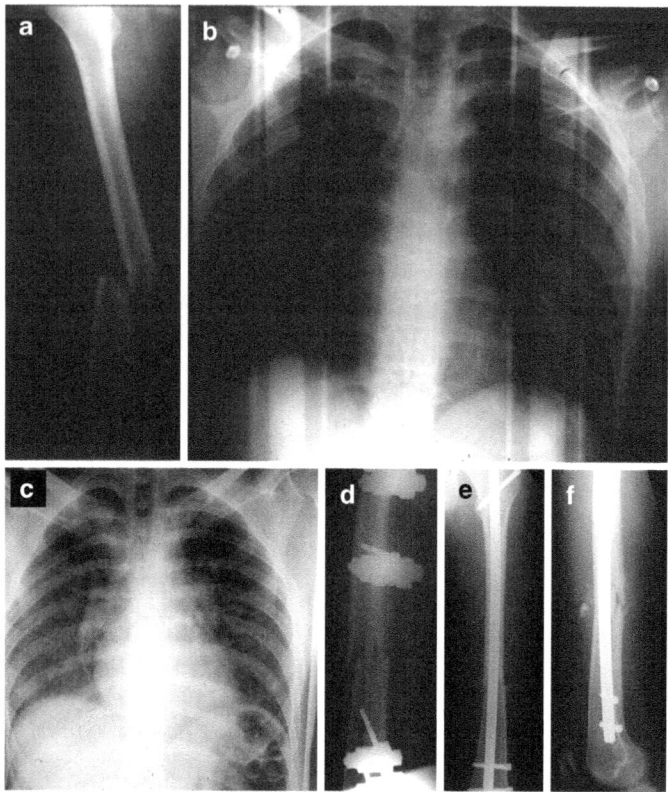

Fig. 3.4 (**a**) AP radiograph of the femur of a 17-year-old male demonstrates oblique fracture through the shaft of the femur. (**b**) AP chest radiograph shows no evidence of lung or chest wall injury. (**c**) AP chest radiograph 4 days later demonstrates diffuse bilateral infiltrates consistent with fat embolism syndrome. (**d**) Anteroposterior radiograph of the femur demonstrates external fixation that was applied in the Intensive Care Unit, and improved alignment of the bone. (**e**) Anteroposterior and (**f**) lateral radiographs of the femur after intramedullary nailing was performed demonstrate proper alignment and stable fixation of the fracture

This is a complex disorder which overlaps Adult Respiratory Distress Syndrome in many ways but is more common in patients with long bone fractures without lung injury. The motion at the unstabilized fracture releases fat into the venous circulation, which can obstruct pulmonary vessels and alter the perfusion of the lung. Additionally, inflammatory mediators are released which alter the permeability of the lung and decrease oxygenation. In young healthy patients, an early symptom of hypoxia is mental status change or confusion. In addition to checking the patient's oxygen saturation, evaluation for delayed presentation of an intracranial injury must be performed.

Other signs and symptoms that are consistent with fat embolism syndrome are tachypnea/shortness of breath, tachycardia, and petechial hemorrhages.

Figure 3.4c is the chest X-ray taken on the fourth day. It depicts diffuse bilateral infiltrates, similar to the radiographic findings in ARDS. The patient was transported by helicopter to the regional trauma center.

What can be done to treat fat embolism syndrome?

The patient experiencing fat embolism syndrome requires oxygen and often ventilatory support. Often, intubation and mechanical ventilation is required. Additionally, improved stabilization of the femur will decrease the release of mediators and fat emboli. The dilemma is that surgery to perform intramedullary nailing of the fracture will increase the release of fat and mediators from the femur during the reaming and insertion of the nail, and the patient may not be stable enough to safely tolerate the transportation to the operating room and the surgery.

In this case, an external fixator was applied to the femur in the Intensive Care Unit (Fig. 3.4d). This provided improved fracture stability without the additional risks of reaming and intramedullary nailing [3]. Three days later, the patient had improved dramatically and had stable respiration and no confusion. Intramedullary nailing of the fracture was performed in the operating room without incident (Fig. 3.4e, f). He went on to a complete recovery and 3 months later walked across the stage to receive his high school diploma on schedule.

The best treatment for fat embolism syndrome and ARDS is prevention [4]. Early stabilization of long bone fractures has become the standard for patients who are stable enough to tolerate surgery [5]. In general, femoral shaft fractures should be surgically stabilized within 24 h. If the patient is too unstable to tolerate major surgery, "damage control" surgery using external fixation can be performed and will decrease the respiratory complications in these patients.

References

1. American College of Surgeons Committee on Trauma. Advanced trauma life support: student course manual. 10th ed. Chicago: American College of Surgeons; 2018.
2. Willett K, Al-Khateeb H, Kotnis R, Bouamra O, Lecky F. Risk of mortality: the relationship with associated injuries and fracture treatment methods in patients with unilateral or bilateral femoral shaft fractures. J Trauma. 2010;69(2):405–10. https://doi.org/10.1097/TA.0b013e3181e6138a.
3. Rothberg DL, Makarewich CA. Fat embolism and fat embolism syndrome. J Am Acad Orthop Surg. 2019;27(8):e346–55. https://doi.org/10.5435/JAAOS-D-17-00571.
4. Nowotarski PJ, Turen CH, Brumback RJ, Scarboro JM. Conversion of external fixation to intramedullary nailing for fractures of the shaft of the femur in multiply injured patients. J Bone Joint Surg Am. 2000;82(6):781–8.
5. Ricci WM, Gallagher B, Haidukewych GJ. Intramedullary nailing of femoral shaft fractures: current concepts. J Am Acad Orthop Surg. 2009;17(5):296–305. https://doi.org/10.5435/00124635-200905000-00004.

Open Fractures

4

A 24-year-old male sustains a severe injury to his left leg when he is struck by a coal car. Clinical photographs depict a 15-cm contaminated open wound (Fig. 4.1) and radiographs depict a comminuted tibial shaft fracture. What are the potential complications of this injury?

This patient has a severe open tibia fracture. Several complications can occur from these injuries. The first and perhaps most critical is significant hemorrhage. Whereas closed tibial fractures can be expected to bleed 1–2 units (500–1000 ml) of blood, an open fracture can bleed much more [1]. An estimate of the amount of blood lost at the scene by the early responders is helpful in triage and in early resuscitation efforts.

Additionally, open fractures are more likely to be associated with vascular injury, neurologic injury, and compartment syndrome than closed fractures. Early and repeated evaluation of pulses, perfusion, neurologic and motor function, and compartment tightness/pressure is essential to diagnose and treat these limb-threatening injuries properly.

The presence of the open wound also makes the chance of infection in the soft tissues and bone (osteomyelitis) much more likely to occur [2] (Fig. 4.2). Additionally, the increased damage to the tissue around the bone, in combination with the contamination and higher risk of infection in open fractures, makes failure of fracture healing (nonunion) more likely to occur.

© The Author(s), under exclusive license to Springer Nature Switzerland AG 2024
J. T. Gorczyca, *Orthopaedic Emergencies*,
https://doi.org/10.1007/978-3-031-62011-9_4

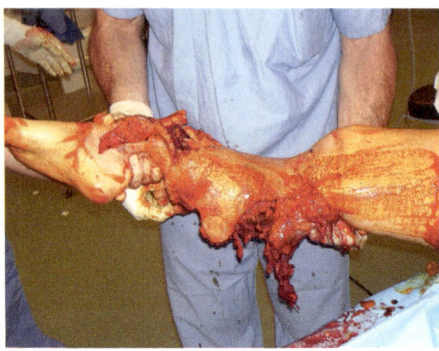

Fig. 4.1 Clinical photograph of pedestrian who sustained a severe open tibia fracture when struck by a car. The open wound and contamination of the tissue place the patient at a higher risk of significant blood loss as well as infection and nonunion of the fracture

Fig. 4.2 Clinical photograph demonstrates an open infected wound extending to the bone (dark area in center of wound) in a patient who had an open tibia fracture 6 months earlier. The fracture has not yet healed

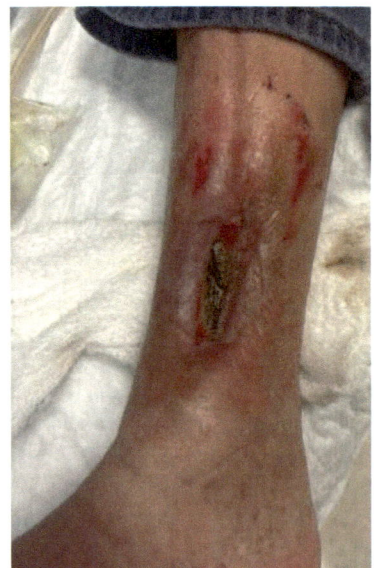

What can be done to minimize the risk of infection in open fractures?

The single most important step that can be taken to minimize the risk of infection is early administration of prophylactic intravenous (IV) antibiotics. The standard is to have IV antibiotics administered within 1 h of arrival in the emergency room, but if these can be given during transport without delaying the patient's arrival, that is even better. Generally, a first generation cephalosporin (e.g., cephalexin) is administered to cover gram-positive organisms, but larger wounds should also be treated with prophylactic coverage for gram-negative bacteria, for example, with gentamicin or ciprofloxacin. Farm injuries and those with potential fecal contamination should also have prophylactic coverage for anaerobic bacteria, such as with penicillin or clindamycin.

The fracture should be straightened/realigned by gentle traction and splinted in a reduced position. The wound should be covered with a sterile gauze or an antibiotic dressing. Photographs of the wound before application of the dressing can be stored in the patient's chart for easy review by others who will treat the patient. The patient should be prepared for surgery as expeditiously as possible.

There is general belief that the earlier the open fracture wound is surgically debrided and irrigated, the lower the rate of infection will be. However, the patient must be thoroughly evaluated for other significant injuries and must be stable enough to tolerate surgery and anesthesia before being taken to the operating room for open fracture surgery [1].

Why is bone infection such a serious problem?

Bone infection (osteomyelitis) is a serious problem because it is difficult to eradicate the bacteria that cause the infection, and the bacteria can lay dormant in an area of poorly vascularized bone (sequestrum) or on surgical implants for months or years before they become active and cause infection (Fig. 4.3). Thus, treatment of infected bone requires debridement of devitalized bone and soft tissue, removal of surgical implants (when possible) and long term (i.e., >6 weeks) intravenous antibiotics. Long term treatment of bone infection is less successful than shorter term

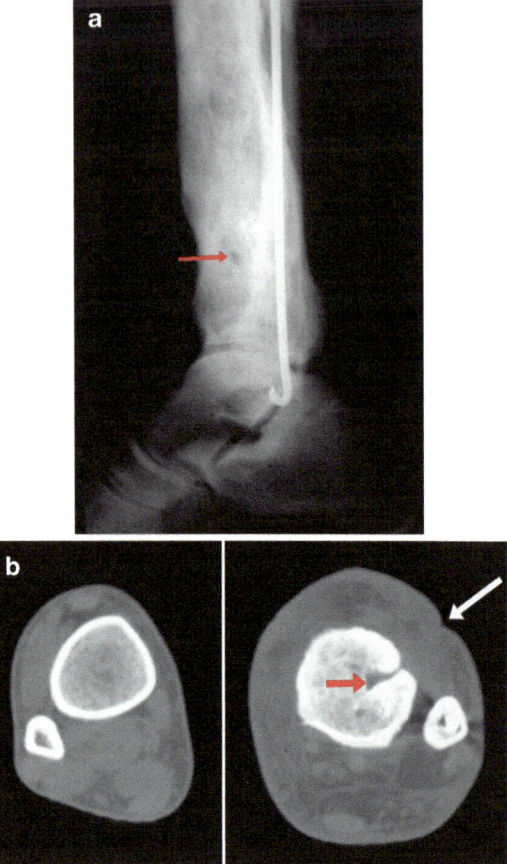

Fig. 4.3 (**a**) Lateral radiograph of the leg demonstrates radiolucent area in bone surrounded by radiodense bone (red arrow). (**b**) Axial CT scan demonstrates radiolucent region (red arrow) that is surrounded almost completely by dense reactive bone and communicates with the subcutaneous tissue drains to the skin (white arrow). The area in the midst contains avascular necrotic debris and infection that cannot be eradicated by the patient's immune defenses and antibiotics. Surgical debridement and long term ($\geq$6 weeks) antibiotics are required to treat this infection, and the chances of success are lower with bone infection than with soft-tissue infections

antibiotics when used for treating soft tissue infections. Also, infection of bone makes the fracture less likely to heal, which will have significant functional consequences for the patient. The important point is that it is better to prevent bone infection than to treat infection.

What is the purpose of surgery for open fractures?

Surgery for open fractures is performed to debride devitalized tissue that if left in place will serve as a nidus from which infection will occur [2]. After debridement, the wound is copiously irrigated with saline or lactated Ringers solution to dilute any microscopic debris and bacteria from the initial contamination. Next, the fracture is aligned (reduced) and stabilized with internal or external fixation. Based on the initial appearance of the wound, the appearance of the wound a few days after initial treatment, and overall clinical judgment, the treating orthopedist may decide to perform repeat irrigation and debridement 2–3 days later to decrease the chance of infection occurring. This may be repeated more often for severe wounds that do not appear to be healing well before closure of the wound is performed [3].

Placement of a foreign body such as a plate or intramedullary rod in a wound could increase the risk of infection (Fig. 4.4). Why is fracture fixation with plate or intramedullary rod performed in open fractures?

Many major studies have been performed comparing the infection rate of open fractures stabilized with internal fixation to those that were not operatively stabilized initially, and there is strong support that early internal fixation of open fractures results in a seemingly *paradoxical* lower rate of infection. The best explanation for this seemingly counterintuitive finding is that the benefits that are achieved by stabilizing the bone, including a stable environment for tissue healing, minimization of bleeding and swelling, and improved immune response—outweigh the disadvantages of placing a foreign body in the wound, and thus the infection rate is lower after internal fixation of open fractures.

Occasionally after open fractures, there is tissue loss that is treated by taking skin from another part of the body and grafting it over the tissue defect. Figure 4.5 shows a patient who had an open fracture of the distal radius in whom the

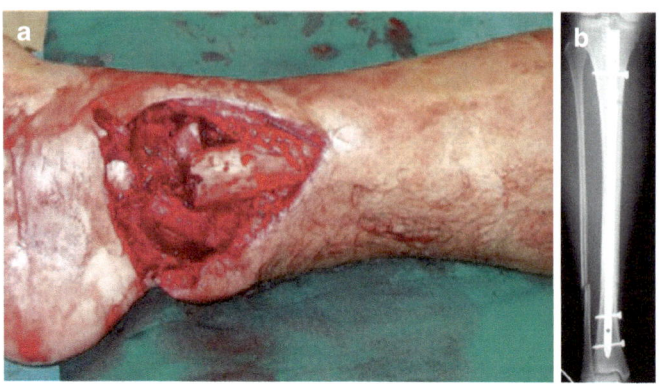

Fig. 4.4 (**a**) Clinical photograph of a patient with a displaced open distal tibia shaft fracture. (**b**) Postoperative AP radiograph of the tibia shows good alignment of the bone with an intramedullary rod in place

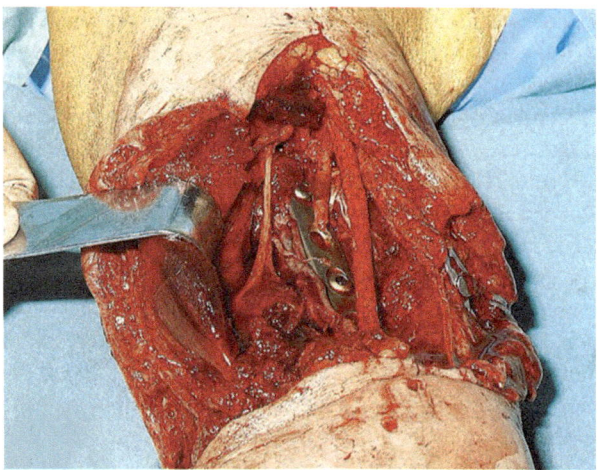

Fig. 4.5 Intraoperative photograph of patient with a severe volar forearm injury that has soft tissue loss with insufficient tissue to cover the exposed bone, nerve, tendon, artery, and metallic plate. Each of those alone would justify a procedure to transfer healthy tissue from another part of the body (i.e., "flap") to cover these structures before skin grafting

skin edges could not be closed. Can you explain why he would not be a good candidate for skin grafting over the wound?

Skin grafting heals best over healthy muscle or subcutaneous tissue/fat. This picture demonstrates exposed nerve, tendon, bone, vessels, and metallic fixation device, none of which are suitable surfaces on which to place skin graft. For this reason, this wound is best treated by moving muscle and or subcutaneous tissue from another part of the body over those surfaces, and grafting skin on top of the transposed tissue. If the muscle and subcutaneous tissue can be moved to this area without disrupting its blood supply, this procedure is referred to as a rotational flap. If muscle must be taken from a distant area, tissue viability requires anastomosis (connection) of its blood vessels to vessels in this area; this procedure is referred to as a free muscle transfer flap [4] ("free flap").

What if a multiply injured patient is not stable enough for a lengthy operation, what should be done?

Many patients are not stable enough to undergo timely surgery for complex fractures and wounds. If the patient can tolerate a brief period of surgery, then limited debridement and perhaps provisional stabilization of fractures with external fixation can be performed. This concept, which is termed "damage control" is used in many types of trauma and follows the principle that limited, provisional intervention that reduces complication risk by providing some fracture stability without significantly compromising the patient's overall health is in the patient's best interest. Once the patient becomes more stable, further surgery can be performed to achieve definitive stabilization of the fracture.

References

1. American College of Surgeons Committee on Trauma. Advanced trauma life support: student course manual. 10th ed. Chicago: American College of Surgeons; 2018.
2. Goldman AH, Tetsworth K. AAOS clinical practice guideline summary: prevention of surgical site infection after major extremity trauma. J Am

Acad Orthop Surg. 2023;31(1):e1–8. https://doi.org/10.5435/JAAOS-D-22-00792. Epub 2022 Nov 3.
3. Weitz-Marshall AD, Bosse MJ. Timing of closure of open fractures. J Am Acad Orthop Surg. 2002;10(6):379–84. https://doi.org/10.5435/00124635-200211000-00001.
4. DeBaun MR, Goodnough LH, Hidden KA, Nork SE, Kleweno CP, Hebert-Davies J. Type III open tibia fractures treated with single-stage immediate medullary nailing and attempted primary closure yield low rates of flap coverage. J Am Acad Orthop Surg. 2023;31(5):252–7. https://doi.org/10.5435/JAAOS-D-22-00469. Epub 2022 Dec 9.

Fractures with Vascular Injuries

5

A 56-year-old intoxicated male falls down a flight of stairs and complains of severe pain just proximal to the left knee? There are no other injuries detected on ATLS evaluation. What should be done to evaluate the leg?

The patient's extremity must undergo thorough examination. After completely disrobing the patient, the skin is visually inspected for contusions, swelling, and color. Any area that has sign of injury should be evaluated with X-rays. If the skin appears grayish, dark, or "dusky", this is consistent with compromised circulation [1]. The patient should then be asked to move the extremity, starting with lifting the leg off of the bed, flexing and extending the knee through as much motion as their comfort will allow, and moving the ankle and toes into flexion and extension/dorsiflexion. Often, with significant injury, the patient will have too much pain to voluntarily move the extremity, and their decision to avoid motion must be respected. However, examination for sensation to light touch in all dermatomes and presence of at least some contraction/motor function of the quadriceps, tibialis anterior, gastroc/soleus, and toe flexors and extensors should be confirmed.

Next, palpation of pulses of the femoral artery at the groin, popliteal artery at the posterior knee, dorsalis pedis artery at the dorsal foot, and posterior tibial artery just posterior to the medial malleolus should be performed. Occasionally, the peroneal artery can be palpated at the anterolateral aspect of the distal leg. If the

© The Author(s), under exclusive license to Springer Nature Switzerland AG 2024
J. T. Gorczyca, *Orthopaedic Emergencies*,
https://doi.org/10.1007/978-3-031-62011-9_5

pulses of these arteries are not palpable (which could be due to excessive soft tissue or hypotension), then they should be evaluated with a Doppler instrument. Capillary refill in the skin should be less than 3 seconds, and any delay is indicative of impaired perfusion.

Patients with significant soft tissue swelling due to the trauma or due to reperfusion after ischemia may develop increased pressure in one of the muscular compartments of the thigh or leg. Elevated compartment pressure can occur from bleeding within a compartment as well. This is especially concerning because many patients are on therapeutic anticoagulants and are at higher risk for significant hemorrhage, even with relatively minor soft tissue injuries. Compartment syndrome should be diagnosed as quickly as possible is order that surgical decompression of the compartment can be performed expediently in order to maintain muscle viability and nerve function. The clinical findings that would indicate compartment syndrome are pain, tight compartments on physical exam, discomfort with passive stretch of the muscles in the compartment, and decreased ability to use/contract the muscles in the compartment. It is important to emphasize that compartment syndrome can occur with open fractures, and that the pulses of arteries which pass through the compartment are often normal despite the compartment syndrome. Compartment syndrome can occur early after injury or it may develop slowly and not occur for a day or two, so repeated evaluation of the extremity is necessary. If there is any doubt of whether or not compartment syndrome is present, the patient should be transferred to a trauma center where fasciotomies can be performed if needed, and measurements of the compartment pressures can be taken to clarify the clinical situation.

If the patient has weak pulses and a fracture is present, the fracture should be aligned/reduced in order to take pressure of the soft tissues and because occasionally this will restore flow through an artery that has been twisted or kinked by the deformity in the leg. If this turns out to be the case, then the fracture should be urgently reduced and stabilized in the operating room in order to maintain alignment of the extremity and perfusion through the vessel.

If the patient has decreased arterial flow and the perfusion does not improve with reduction of the extremity, what should be done next?

The next step would be to obtain an arteriogram or a CT angiogram in order to establish the location of the arterial injury and plan a bypass procedure or excision of the thrombus to restore perfusion to the extremity [2]. The Vascular Surgery team should be notified as early as possible about a potential arterial injury. The arteries of the entire extremity should be viewed angiographically to assure that there are not two different levels of injury, as both injuries would have to be addressed.

If there is concern for a vascular injury and a vascular surgeon is not available at the medical center, then the patient should be transported to a trauma center as soon as they are medically stable enough to tolerate the transportation [1].

X-rays show that the patient has a proximal tibia fracture and the arteriogram shows arterial occlusion at the same level. Which should be treated first, the arterial injury or the fracture?

It is important to fix the arterial injury as quickly as possible in order to prevent necrosis and maintain function of the extremity. Generally, a limb can tolerate 4–6 h of warm ischemia before irreversible changes to the tissues occur, so there is limited time to make a decision and perform surgery [1].

However, if the bone can be stabilized quickly, this can make it easier for the vascular surgeon to perform the repair, and the femur will be at the correct length and stable, which will facilitate the surgery. Additionally, if the arterial repair is performed first, there is a chance that the repair will be traumatized by the manipulation of the femur during the bony procedure. Thus, the question of which procedure should be done first is generally a judgment call to be made by the vascular surgeon. If they believe that there is enough time to perform expedient stabilization of the bone first, whether by internal stabilization or external fixation, then that should be performed first (Fig. 5.1). If time is limited and irreversible ischemia is looming, then they will decide to perform vascular repair first, knowing that there is a chance that revision of the repair could become necessary after the bony stabilization is performed.

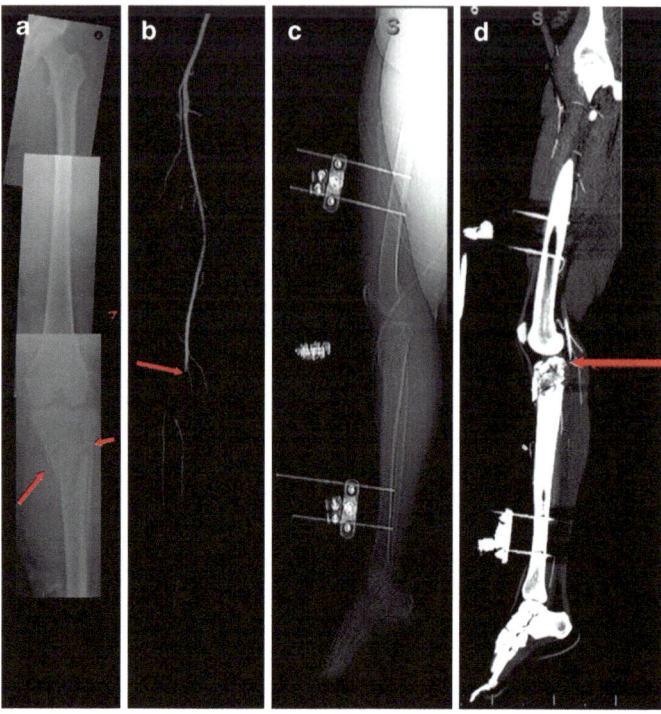

Fig. 5.1 (**a**) Composite anteroposterior radiographs of lower extremity demonstrate oblique fracture of proximal tibia (red arrows). (**b**) CT reconstruction of arteriogram depicts disruption of arterial flow near the branching of the superficial femoral artery to the tibioperoneal trunk and anterior tibial artery (red arrow). (**c**) Lateral radiograph demonstrates fracture in good alignment with external fixation. (**d**) Arteriogram after external fixation shows location of vascular occlusion at proximal tibia fracture (red arrow), emphasizing that fractures can be associated with neurovascular injuries caused by the force of the initial trauma

References

1. Halvorson JJ, Anz A, Langfitt M, Deonanan JK, Scott A, Teasdall RD, Carroll EA. Vascular injury associated with extremity trauma: initial diagnosis and management. J Am Acad Orthop Surg. 2011;19(8):495–504. https://doi.org/10.5435/00124635-201108000-00005.
2. American College of Surgeons Committee on Trauma. Advanced trauma life support: student course manual. 10th ed. Chicago: American College of Surgeons; 2018.

Pediatric Supracondylar Humerus Fractures

6

An 8-year-old girl falls from a swing onto her outstretched hand and has immediate pain and deformity of the arm. She is taken to the hospital where she is noted to have good perfusion of the skin. X-rays are obtained (Fig. 6.1). What is the mechanism that causes this injury and why is this injury common in children but not in adults?

This fracture is caused by a hyperextension force on the elbow which occurs when the child reaches their arm out to stop a fall. Children are more active than adults, they have elbows that hyperextend more than those of adults, and the elbow capsule in children is comparatively stronger than in adults. Thus, children usually sustain a fracture when they fall and the elbow is forcibly hyperextended, causing the olecranon process to collide with and bend the olecranon fossa of the humerus, which fractures the bone. In adults, the elbow joint capsule is comparatively weaker than the bone, so a hyperextension force is more likely to result in tear of the capsule and a posterior elbow dislocation.

The child's parents inform you that they would like to achieve an excellent outcome without having surgical intervention. What is a potential complication of nonoperative treatment of this injury?

The elbow is an unforgiving joint, and fractures in the elbow region that heal with deformity are likely to result in functional or cosmetic impairment. The challenge with this fracture is that it is

© The Author(s), under exclusive license to Springer Nature Switzerland AG 2024
J. T. Gorczyca, *Orthopaedic Emergencies*,
https://doi.org/10.1007/978-3-031-62011-9_6

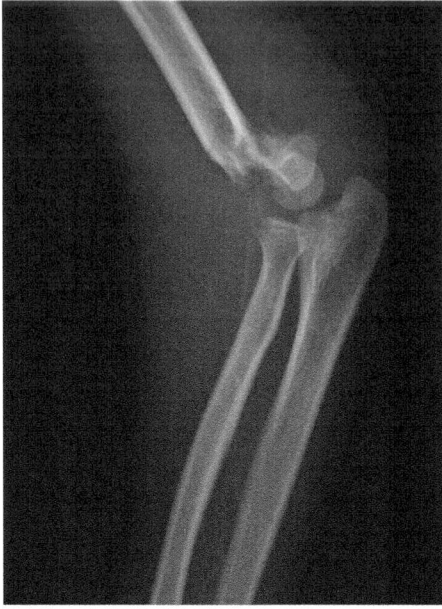

Fig. 6.1 Anteroposterior radiograph of the upper extremity of an 8-year-old child who fell off a swing set and sustained this markedly displaced supracondylar humerus fracture

unstable and likely to continually displace after reduction, even when immobilized. The most stable position in which to maintain long-term reduction of the fracture is with elbow hyperflexion. The problem with that positioning is that with the acutely injured elbow, the swelling is likely to increase for a couple of days, which in combination with elbow hyperflexion (which will decrease perfusion of the tissues as well as venous return from the forearm) is likely to result in compartment syndrome of the forearm muscles. Undiagnosed or untreated compartment syndrome will result in Volkmann's ischemic contracture of the forearm and complete or significant loss of hand function (Fig. 6.2).

In most cases, a displaced pediatric supracondylar humerus fracture can be reduced with closed methods in the operating

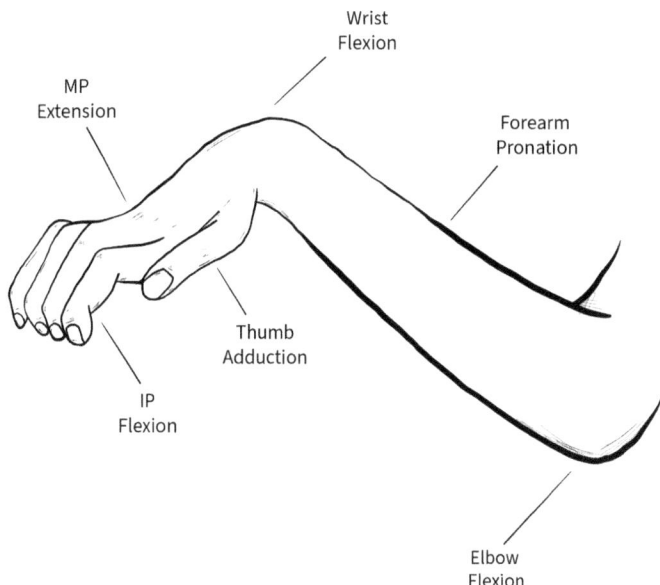

Wrist
Flexion

MP
Extension

Forearm
Pronation

Thumb
Adduction

IP
Flexion

Elbow
Flexion

Fig. 6.2 Drawing illustrates the devastating long-term outcome of forearm compartment syndrome, which is more common when pediatric supracondylar humerus fractures are treated with closed reduction and immobilization in flexion. (Drawing courtesy of Louis C. Okafor, MD)

room, and then held in this position with two or more wires placed percutaneously (Fig. 6.3). The reduction of the fracture is now more stable and is maintained well enough by the wires that the elbow can be positioned in a neutral position (i.e., 90° flexion) that optimizes distal perfusion and venous outflow, thereby decreasing the risk of compartment syndrome and Volkmann's ischemic contracture.

What are the early (preoperative) treatment steps in the treatment of the child with a displaced supracondylar humerus fracture?

The extremity should be gently aligned into a straight position with the elbow moderately flexed (approximately 45 degrees) to re-align any kinked or twisted vessels and to reduce pressure on

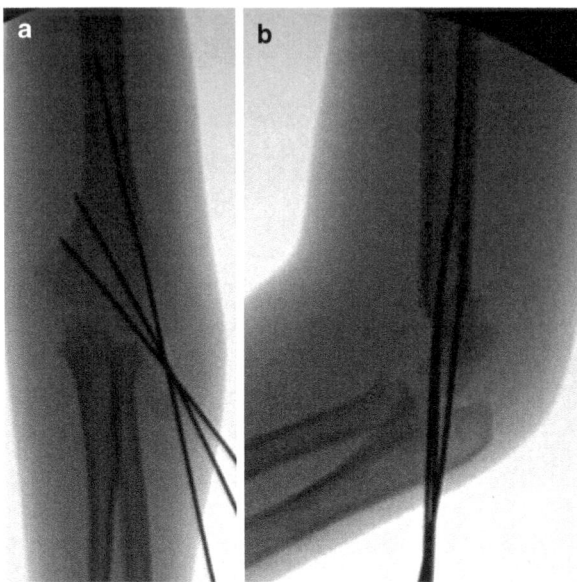

Fig. 6.3 Intraoperative AP (**a**) and lateral (**b**) fluoroscopic images of displaced supracondylar humerus fracture that was treated appropriately with closed reduction and percutaneous fixation

the soft tissues. Attempts at manipulating the arm to improve the reduction of the fracture, however, should not be performed as they are unlikely to result in a stable improvement in fracture alignment, and they will cause further trauma to the soft tissues.

The perfusion of the skin should be evaluated by assessing capillary refill. Pulses should be investigated by palpation and by Doppler ultrasound if they are weak or not palpable. A neurologic examination of the extremity should be performed. Any sign of open wound or pressure/puckering of the skin should be noted. Compromised perfusion, altered neurologic examination, and skin compromise warrant urgent intervention by the orthopedic and in some cases the vascular team.

How soon should displaced pediatric supracondylar humerus fractures be operatively stabilized?

Fractures with vascular impairment, nerve injury, or pressure/puckering of the skin should be reduced and operatively stabilized emergently. Fractures without these pressing conditions can safely wait up to 24 h before surgery [1]. As the neurovascular status of the limb may change and one or more of these indications for emergent surgery can develop any time after injury, it is important to transfer any patient with displaced supracondylar humerus fracture to the appropriate treating facility as soon as possible after injury, and to continue to monitor the physical examination to detect any change as early as possible.

What is the most common nerve injury associated with this fracture?

Any or all of the nerves in the vicinity of the fracture can be injured with a displaced supracondylar humerus fracture. These nerves are the radial nerve, the median nerve, and the ulnar nerve. The most commonly injured is the median nerve, often its anterior interosseous branch. This nerve branch serves the radial half of the flexor digitorum profundus muscle, the entire flexor pollicis longus muscle, and the pronator quadratus muscle. It also provides sensation to the volar surface of digits 2, 3, and 4. This is significant because the nerve injury may not be obvious unless one performs a detailed examination for thumb interphalangeal flexion, index DIP flexion, and long finger sensation at the palmar surface. Fortunately, most of these nerve palsies resolve without treatment, but the early diagnosis is essential in order to be sure that a nerve injury present after surgery was not caused by fracture reduction during which the nerve was injured or trapped in the fracture site.

Postoperatively, the patient's extremity is immobilized in a splint and later in a cast until bridging bone is visible on follow-up radiographs (generally 4–6 weeks after injury, and as with most fractures in children, the younger the child, the sooner the healing). When the fracture is healed, the wires are removed and the patient gradually returns to normal activities. Wire removal is usually performed with the patient awake in the clinic. Children are active enough and heal quickly enough that in the great majority of cases, formal physical therapy is not required after healing of the fracture (Fig. 6.4).

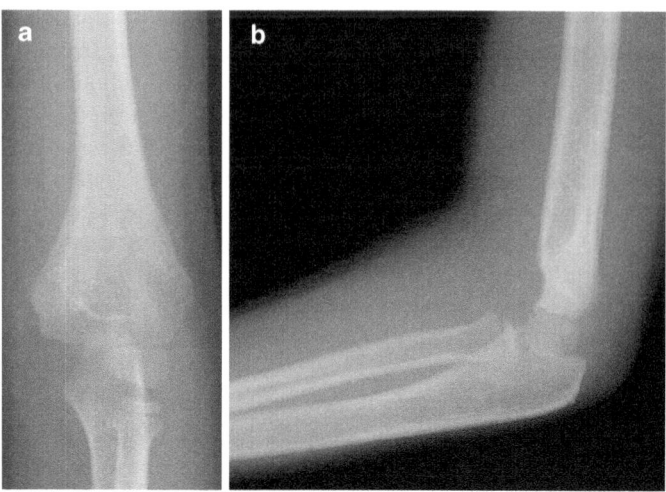

Fig. 6.4 Anteroposterior (**a**) and lateral (**b**) radiographs taken 3 months postoperatively demonstrate excellent healing and alignment

Reference

1. Abzug JM, Herman MJ. Management of supracondylar humerus fractures in children: current concepts. J Am Acad Orthop Surg. 2012;20(2):69–77. https://doi.org/10.5435/JAAOS-20-02-069.

Open Pelvis Fractures

7

A 48-year-old man is run over by a large fork lift and sustains an open pelvis fracture. What is the risk of mortality, and what is the typical cause of mortality?

Open pelvis fractures are often devastating injuries which carry a mortality rate as high as 50% [1]. The injuring force causes progressive deformity and disruption of the pelvis, then further displacement until all of the tissue near the injury is torn from deep to superficial. Thus, occasionally the skin wound is the "tip of the iceberg" and appears relatively benign, whereas the damage to the underlying bone and deep soft-tissues is more severe (Fig. 7.1).

The mechanism and energy causing the open pelvis fracture is usually more violent than those that cause closed fractures, so there will be greater disruption to the blood vessels and consequently more bleeding. Additionally, as with most open fractures, open pelvis fractures tend to allow for more blood loss through the open wound, so the early mortality rate from hemorrhage is significantly higher with open pelvis fractures [2].

Interestingly, patients with these injuries have a bimodal death distribution. Many patients die in the first few minutes, hours, or days from hemorrhage, and then there is a second peak in the mortality rate 5–6 days after injury when overwhelming sepsis from infection of the open wound occurs.

J. T. Gorczyca, *Orthopaedic Emergencies*,
https://doi.org/10.1007/978-3-031-62011-9_7

The patient is resuscitated according to ATLS protocols and as described in Chap. 1. The pelvis is provisionally stabilized with an external device. What can be done to reduce the risk of infection and sepsis?

Like most open fractures, the open pelvis fracture should be treated with early prophylactic antibiotics, operative debridement, and irrigation of the tissues. Often, several operative debridements that are scheduled to occur 2–3 days apart, are necessary to debride tissue that may appear healthy at the first debridement, but progressively becomes less viable with time. Due to the proximity of the open pelvis wound to the lower end of the GI tract (Fig. 7.2), fecal contamination of the wound is likely and prophylactic antibiotics should be directed at gram negative bacteria and anaerobic bacteria in addition to the usual gram positive cocci. Diversion of

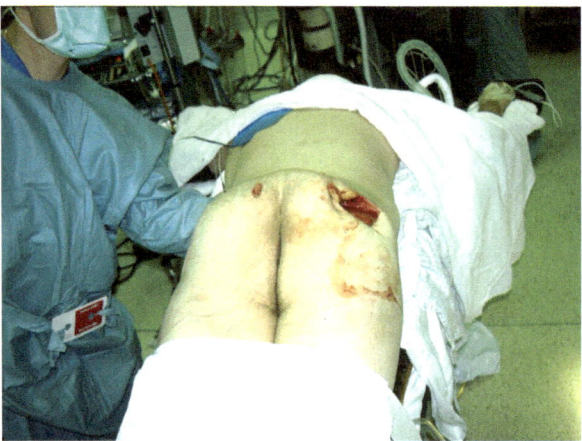

Fig. 7.1 Clinical photograph of patient with open pelvis fracture. The physician's sterile hand is placed inside the wound at the patient's left lateral pelvis, across the completely degloved posterior pelvis, and the fingers can be visualized emerging from a right posterior wound. This emphasizes the point that the injury to deep structures is usually significantly worse than the injury to the superficial structures

the colonic contents to a site farther from the open wound (temporary diverting colostomy) is usually of benefit in minimizing the contamination of the traumatic wound by fecal bacteria [3].

Operative stabilization of the fracture once the wound appears clean and healthy enough to do so is associated with improved comfort and survival, and may have a beneficial impact on infection prevention (Fig. 7.3).

Thus, the open pelvis fracture combines the worst characteristics of open fractures with the worst characteristics of pelvis fractures, and has a mortality risk that is representative of this fact [1, 2]. A multidisciplinary approach to hemodynamic resuscitation, surgical debridement, antibiotic management, ICU care, diverting colostomy, and operative pelvic stabilization is required in order to optimize the chance of survival for patients with these extreme injuries.

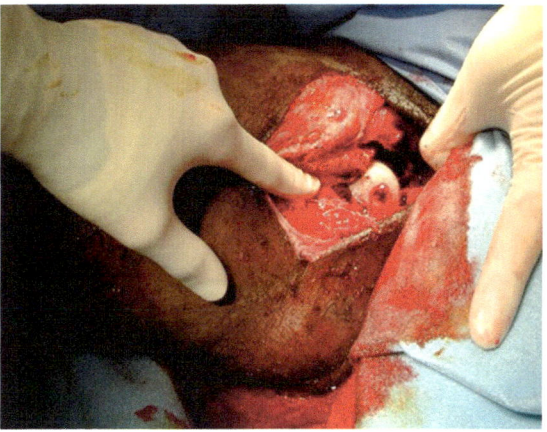

Fig. 7.2 Clinical photograph of a patient with an open pelvis fracture demonstrates the femoral head visualized through the wound in the groin. Diverting colostomy should be performed to decrease any ongoing contamination of the wound from the patient's gastrointestinal tract

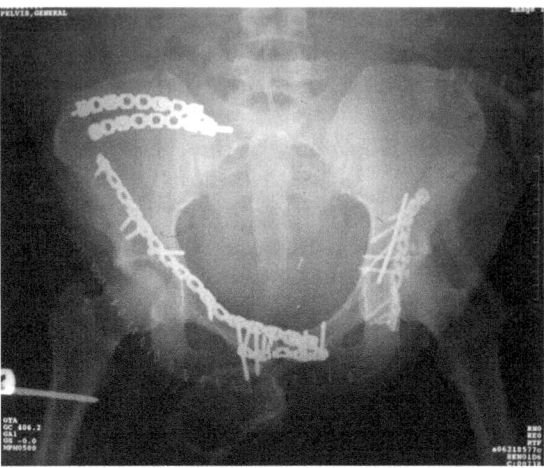

Fig. 7.3 Radiograph of the pelvis after open reduction and internal fixation of open pelvis fracture. Surgical stabilization is performed for the reasons explained in the chapters on pelvis fractures and on open fractures: to improve patient comfort and mobilization, to decrease ongoing hemorrhage, to reduce the risk of infection, to improve healing, and to restore alignment of the pelvis for long-term functional benefit. Definitive surgery, which in this case took more than 8 h to complete, should be performed when the patient's status is optimized enough to allow this

References

1. Jones AL, Powell JN, Kellam JF, McCormack RG, Dust W, Wimmer P. Open pelvic fractures. A multicenter retrospective analysis. Orthop Clin North Am. 1997;28(3):345–50. https://doi.org/10.1016/s0030-5898(05)70293-5.
2. Langford JR, Burgess AR, Liporace FA, Haidukewych GJ. Pelvic fractures: part 1. Evaluation, classification, and resuscitation. J Am Acad Orthop Surg. 2013;21(8):448–57. https://doi.org/10.5435/JAAOS-21-08-448.
3. Fitzgerald CA, Moore TJ Jr, Morse BC, Subramanian A, Dente CJ, Patel DC, Reisman WM, Schenker ML, Gelbard RB. The role of diverting colostomy in traumatic blunt open pelvic fractures. Am Surg. 2017;83(8):e280–2.

Dislocated Joints

8

Figure 8.1 shows the AP pelvis X-ray of a 26-year-old man with severe right hip pain after a front impact motor vehicle collision. What is the injury?

The patient has a *posterior* right hip dislocation. The radiograph demonstrates that the femoral head is no longer centered in the acetabulum, and that the femur is positioned proximally due to the pull of the powerful muscles that cross the hip joint.

Radiographs of a joint should always show two orthogonal (i.e., 90° to each other) views of the joint in order to properly visualize the joint [1]. Some dislocations or subluxations may appear well-positioned on a single X-ray or on two non-orthogonal radiographs. Thus, there is danger of missing the diagnosis and not treating the injury properly if two orthogonal radiographs are not obtained [2].

What are some of the problems caused by dislocated joints?

Joint dislocations can cause many problems due to the displacement at the joint: Nerves and vessels will be stretched by the trauma and will remain under tension or pressure while the joint is dislocated [3]. The cartilage of the joint is often sheared or scraped off of the bone by the traumatic event. The pain from the injury will cause strong muscle contracture that compresses the dislocated articular cartilage against bone or other tissue. Similarly, the dislocated bone can result in pressure on the overlying skin with impaired soft-tissue perfusion and imminent skin necrosis.

© The Author(s), under exclusive license to Springer Nature
Switzerland AG 2024
J. T. Gorczyca, *Orthopaedic Emergencies*,
https://doi.org/10.1007/978-3-031-62011-9_8

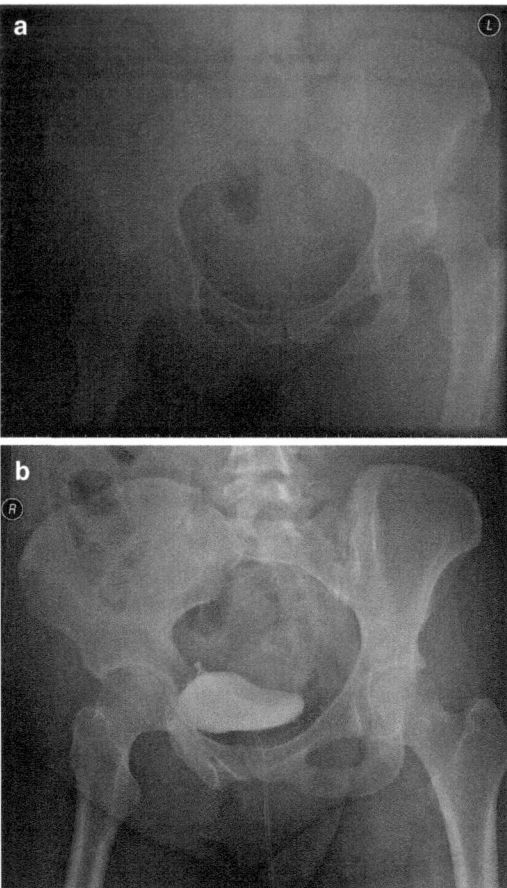

Fig. 8.1 (**a**) AP radiograph of the pelvis demonstrates posterior hip dislocation in patient who was involved in a front impact motor vehicle collision and
was not wearing a seatbelt. (**b**) AP radiograph of the pelvis after successful
closed reduction in the emergent room. Post-reduction CT scan of the pelvis
should be performed to evaluate potential fractures as well as to visualize
intra-articular tissue or bone that could cause joint damage

An additional concern with some dislocations is impaired perfusion of the dislocated bone. This is true with hip dislocations:
the great majority of the blood flow to the dislocated femoral head

comes from arteries that pass from distal to proximal along the femoral neck and capsule to the femoral head (Fig. 8.2). When the hip is dislocated, these vessels may be torn, twisted, kinked or compressed, thereby reducing the perfusion [1].

What can be done to minimize the long-term effects of these problems?

It is believed that urgent reduction of a dislocated hip will realign some of these vessels and restore perfusion to the femoral head before necrosis of the bone can occur. Other benefits of early reduction of the dislocation are improved patient comfort, removal of pressure on the nerves and arteries which need to function distal to the dislocation, and reduction of pressure on the cartilage

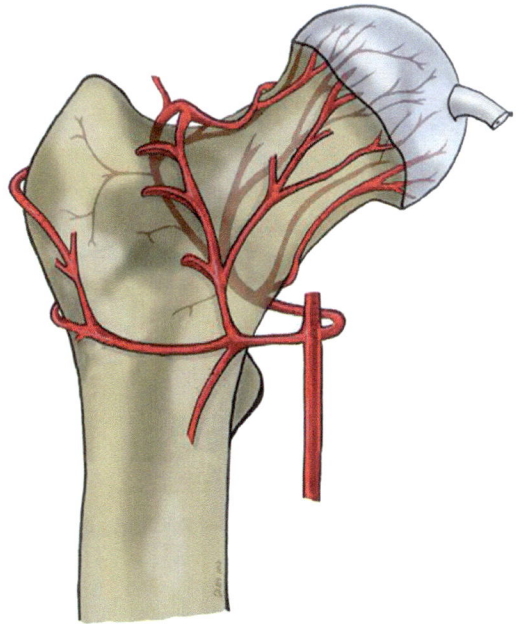

Fig. 8.2 Drawing demonstrates blood supply of femoral head and neck, with branches passing along the neck that are vulnerable to injury when a femoral neck fracture is displaced. The capsule of the hip joint is not included in order to improve visualization of the blood vessels. (Drawing courtesy of Louis C. Okafor, MD)

and skin [3]. Thus, urgent reduction of dislocated joints will be beneficial if the overall condition of the patient is stable enough to tolerate the procedure.

Why is the mechanism that causes most hip dislocations important?

These posterior hip dislocations are usually caused by sudden stop of a motorized vehicle, which causes the driver or passenger's momentum to carry the body forward until the knee strikes the dashboard, stopping the lower extremity while the upper body and pelvis continues forward, resulting in posterior dislocation of the hip, sometimes with a fracture of the acetabulum as well (Fig. 8.3).

There are two reasons why the mechanism that causes hip dislocations is important. First, this mechanism (knee striking dash-

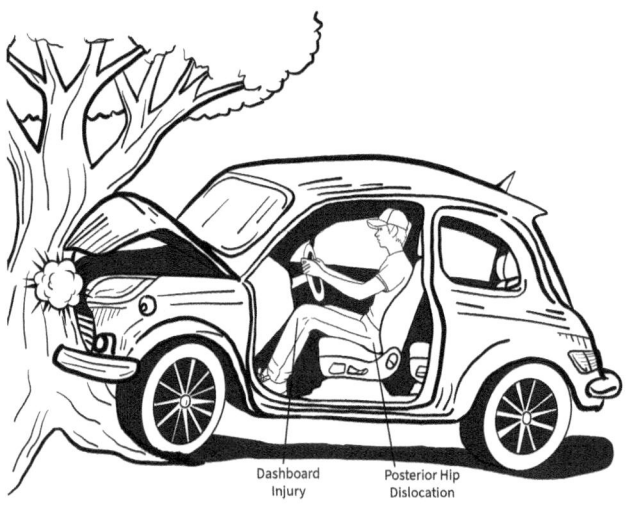

Dashboard   Posterior Hip
Injury   Dislocation

Fig. 8.3 Drawing illustrates the mechanism causing many posterior hip dislocations: knee impact on dashboard caused by sudden stop of quickly moving vehicle, while body that is not properly restrained with a seatbelt continues forward due to considerable momentum. This mechanism can cause knee injury in addition to posterior hip dislocation. (Drawing courtesy of Louis C. Okafor, MD)

board) may also result in distal femur fracture, patella fracture, and other injuries to the knee, which may not be noticed by the patient who is distracted by the pain and displacement of the hip dislocation. Efforts should be taken to examine for any sign of associated knee injury. This underscores the importance of examining the entire patient after significant trauma.

Second, many of these injuries are preventable if the vehicle occupant takes proper precautions, including wearing a seatbelt/restraint which is snug around the lower waist, and positioning the seat as far back as possible while still allowing the driver proper position for control of the accelerator and brake pedals. Airbags are an additional benefit to patient safety, but are not as effective if the vehicle occupant does not also wear a seatbelt.

How is a joint dislocation reduced?

After a thorough neurovascular examination is obtained, the next step is to provide adequate anesthesia before the reduction maneuver. This is especially important for hip dislocations, as the pain caused by the injury will cause the powerful muscles around the hip to contract, thereby making it almost impossible that reduction maneuvers will be successful. Adequate anesthesia is generally achieved with conscious sedation, but intra-articular or regional anesthetic techniques can be helpful. Once the muscles are noted to be relaxed on examination, traction and manipulation is performed. For hip dislocations, the patient is positioned supine and one person should stabilize the pelvis while a second person applies traction to the extremity as the hip is manipulated into flexion, adduction and internal rotation. This usually results in a palpable "clunk" as the femoral head slides into position.

The common anterior dislocation of the glenohumeral (shoulder) joint is likewise reduced best after analgesia and consequent relaxation of muscle contracture. There are several methods of reduction—a common method involves stabilizing the torso while longitudinal traction on the arm is applied with the shoulder mildly abducted, the upper arm is pulled laterally with a sheet, and the arm is rotated internally and externally at the shoulder joint. While reduction of dislocated shoulder joints are commonly performed by Emergency Room physicians in North America, dislocated hip joints should be reduced by Orthopedic Surgeons whenever possible.

What should be done if the dislocated hip cannot be reduced under conscious sedation in the emergency room?

The patient with an irreducible hip should be taken urgently to the operating room. Often, under general anesthesia, the additional muscle relaxation will be sufficient to allow reduction by the same techniques that until now have been unsuccessful. If closed reduction in the operating room is not successful, then an open surgical reduction should be performed to remove any structures that are blocking the reduction.

What are the consequences of compromised blood flow to bone such as the femoral head?

Bone is a living organ that requires blood supply to remodel and repair the microfractures that occur during normal activity. Bone death from lack of blood supply is called avascular necrosis. Occasionally, the necrotic bone will be revitalized by vascular ingrowth and the bone will be restored to normal. If the vascular supply is insufficient, either by traumatic damage to the vessels or due to other physiologic problems, the normal repair of microfractures and revitalization of bone will not occur. With time, the microfractures will eventually become larger fractures. The larger fractures are painful and result in resorption of bone in the femoral head. This may result in collapse of the bone underneath the articular surface (subchondral bone) (Fig. 8.4). The irregular articular surface results in premature wear of the articular cartilage and osteoarthritis, and often the unbearable pain of osteoarthritis. Arthritic pain in the hip can severely compromise a patient's activity level and quality of life.

Are hip replacements good operations?

Hip replacement (arthroplasty) is the elective procedure (of all surgical procedures) that is associated with the greatest improvement in quality of life. Most patients have had progressive pain for years before surgery and are able to return to walking without pain and return to an active lifestyle shortly after the procedure (Fig. 8.5). Unfortunately, the complications of infection, venous thromboembolism, and joint dislocation, although rare, are devas-

Fig. 8.4 Lateral radiograph of hip demonstrates localized resorption of bone in the subchondral region of the femoral head in a patient 18 months after posterior hip dislocation. He had been symptom-free until 6 weeks earlier when he started having vague thigh pain, which is not an unusual symptom for avascular necrosis of the femoral head

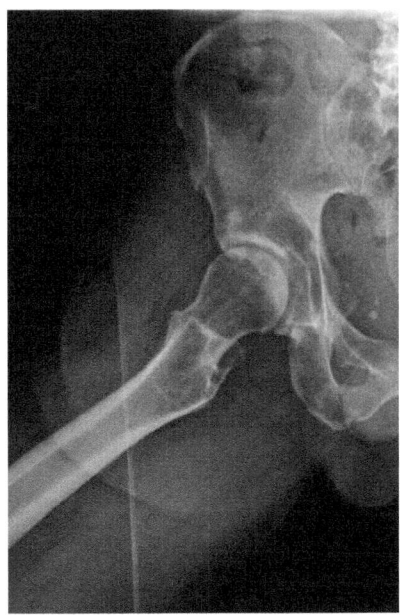

tating problems to those who must endure them. Additionally, the average expectancy for functional hip arthroplasty is between 15 and 25 years, so even when the procedure performs well, young and middle aged persons are likely to require a revision procedure (or two or more revisions) at some point in their lifetime, and the complications of revision arthroplasty are worse those of primary arthroplasty [4].

In summary, joint dislocations are associated with multiple complications that increase in likelihood with the duration of dislocation, so expedient reduction of a dislocated joint is the standard. The complication of avascular necrosis of the hip can be treated with hip arthroplasty, but if the patient's native femoral head survives the dislocation, it will function better than a hip replacement. Thus, efforts should be directed toward timely reduction of the dislocation in an attempt to avoid arthroplasty if possible.

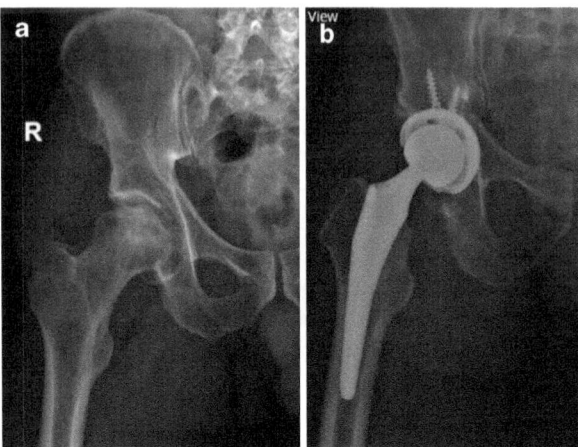

Fig. 8.5 (**a**) AP radiograph of the hip 3 years after posterior hip dislocation treated with closed reduction demonstrates irregular shape of femoral head and sclerosis in the femoral head. (**b**) Total hip arthroplasty was performed to alleviate the chronic pain and to improve activity level. Unfortunately, most hip replacements will loosen and become symptomatic with time. Thus, while it is a very effective procedure, the risks must be weighed against the benefits before undertaking this major procedure

References

1. Foulk DM, Mullis BH. Hip dislocation: evaluation and management. J Am Acad Orthop Surg. 2010;18(4):199–209. https://doi.org/10.5435/00124635-201004000-00003.
2. Youm T, Takemoto R, Park BK. Acute management of shoulder dislocations. J Am Acad Orthop Surg. 2014;22(12):761–71. https://doi.org/10.5435/JAAOS-22-12-761.
3. Mook WR, Ligh CA, Moorman CT, Leversedge FJ. Nerve injury complicating multiligament knee injury: current concepts and treatment algorithm. J Am Acad Orthop Surg. 2013;21(6):343–54. https://doi.org/10.5435/JAAOS-21-06-343.
4. Evans JT, Evans JP, Walker RW, Blom AW, Whitehouse MR, Sayers A. How long does a hip replacement last? A systematic review and meta-analysis of case series and national registry reports with more than 15 years of follow-up. Lancet. 2019;393(10172):647–54. https://doi.org/10.1016/S0140-6736(18)31665-9. Epub 2019 Feb 14. PMID: 30782340; PMCID: PMC6376618.

Septic Joints

9

A patient has a swollen right knee that started hurting 2 days ago without any inciting event. She has had a low-grade fever, has pain with walking, and has exacerbation of her pain with knee motion (Fig. 9.1). The skin around the knee is warm. X-rays of the knee are normal. What is the likely diagnosis?

This patient appears to have a septic knee joint. Other findings on evaluation might include inguinal adenopathy, chills, and elevated white blood cell count, CRP, and erythrocyte sedimentation rate [1–3]. Some patients will have a history of a previous knee infection, recent upper respiratory or urinary tract infection, previous surgery in the knee area, or penetrating injury to the joint.

What else is in the differential diagnosis?

Other common causes of a non-traumatic, swollen painful knee include synovitis of the knee, gout/pseudogout, viral arthritis, rheumatoid arthritis, Lyme disease, and osteoarthritis.

Why is it important to establish the diagnosis of septic joint as early as possible?

Bacterial infections in joints cause the release of chemicals that are destructive to joint cartilage. The bacteria can continue to survive and the chemicals may continue to damage the joint cartilage and bone until the joint is surgically irrigated and debrided of devitalized tissue (Fig. 9.2). Without surgical intervention, intravenous antibiotics alone are unlikely to eradicate the bacteria and

J. T. Gorczyca, *Orthopaedic Emergencies*,
https://doi.org/10.1007/978-3-031-62011-9_9

Fig. 9.1 Clinical photograph demonstrates swollen knee in patient without a history of injury. Infected (i.e., septic) joint must be ruled out

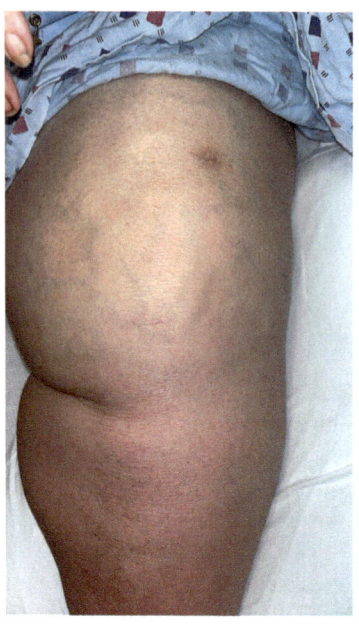

stop the damage, so early diagnosis, surgical treatment, and antibiotics is the standard of care [2].

Occasionally, it may be difficult to establish the diagnosis of septic knee based on symptoms, physical examination, and laboratory tests. Can you think of any patients who may have less impressive examination and laboratory findings despite the fact that they have an active bacterial joint infection?

Patients who are immunocompromised, immunosuppressed, or diabetic may have fewer symptoms of infection and are at risk for being under-evaluated and mis-diagnosed as uninfected. Additionally, patients who have recently received antibiotics, either for the suspected joint infection or for another infection, are more likely to have unimpressive examination and laboratory findings due to the fact that the bacteria have been somewhat suppressed and there is less of an inflammatory response [1]. In these cases, further tests are warranted. Radiographs of the joint may

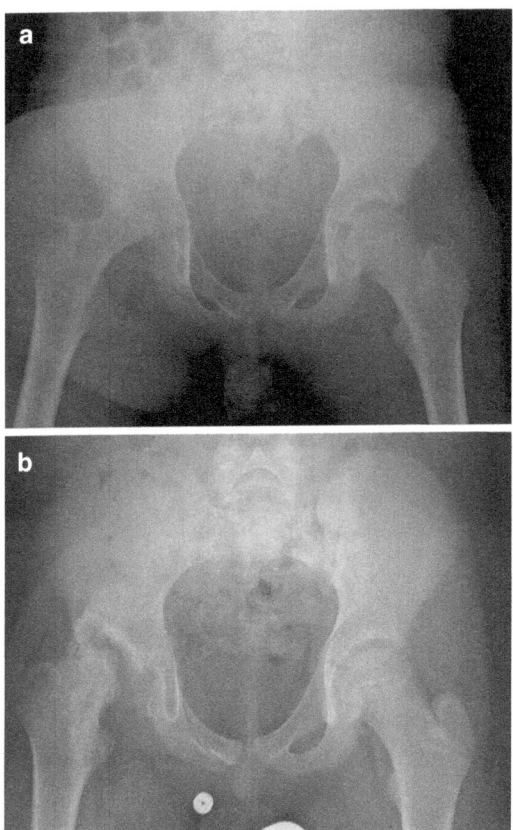

Fig. 9.2 (**a**) AP pelvis radiograph demonstrates destruction of bone at femoral head caused by previously mis-diagnosed and untreated septic joint. (**b**) Radiograph 1 year later demonstrates more severe destruction of bone, with deformity and displacement. It is essential to establish the diagnosis of septic joint and to initiate treatment as soon as possible in order to prevent such a dreadful complication

reveal fluid or gas in the joint. A CT scan or MRI may also be helpful to evaluate for fluid or air in the joint in cases in which the radiographs are equivocal but the clinical findings are suggestive of septic joint (Fig. 9.3).

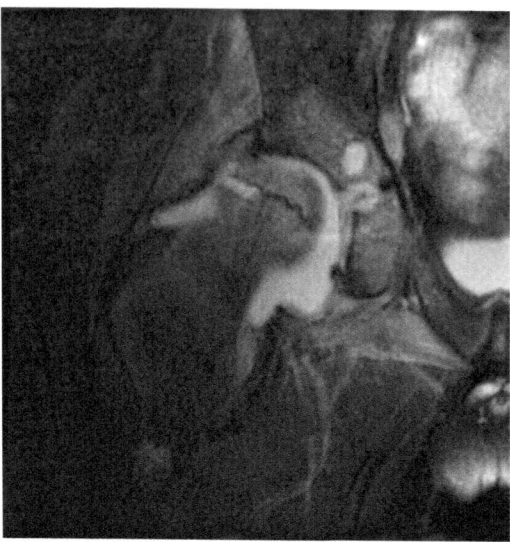

Fig. 9.3 MRI scan demonstrates abundant fluid in hip joint which is consistent with septic hip joint, and warrants aspiration of the fluid for cell count and culture, or based on clinical findings, urgent surgical debridement. CT scan and ultrasound studies can also be used to detect fluid in a joint

If physical examination or radiographic study demonstrates that there is fluid in the joint, what should be done to establish the diagnosis?

When in doubt, needle aspiration of the involved joint fluid will be helpful in making the diagnosis of septic joint (Fig. 9.4). The ankle, knee, elbow, wrist, and shoulder can be easily aspirated based on palpation of the anatomy. Aspiration of the hip joint can also be performed based on palpation but is more accurately performed if ultrasound or CT guidance of the aspiration needle is used to assure that the correct location is aspirated. The fluid that is obtained should be sent for nucleated cell count, gram stain, and culture. A septic joint typically has >50,000 nucleated cells per microliter. A gram stain may demonstrate bacteria, but the gram stain sometimes shows no bacteria even in patients with florid septic joint.

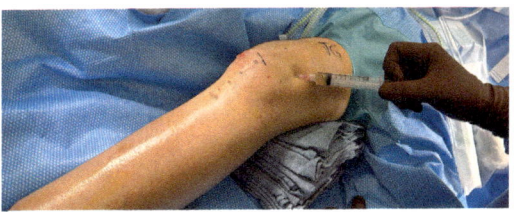

Fig. 9.4 Needle aspiration of joint, performed under sterile technique, can be used to obtain joint fluid for further analysis in order to establish the diagnosis of infection

What bacteria is most likely to be isolated in culture?

Staphylococcus aureus is the bacteria which most commonly causes septic arthritis [3]. It is also the bacteria which most commonly cause other orthopedic infections. Interestingly, 36% of aspirates taken from infected joints do not grow bacteria on culture in the microbiology lab. The reason for this high negative culture rate is likely multifactorial: e.g., fastidious organisms, imperfect technique, and/or the effect of any antibiotics that may have been administered.

What is the postoperative course for a patient with a septic joint?

After surgical irrigation and debridement of an infected joint, the patient should be treated with intravenous antibiotics until there is definite improvement in the patient's comfort, temperature, and laboratory findings, at which point the patient may be transitioned to oral antibiotics for another week or two. The details of treatment and the choice of antibiotics should be made by a specialist in Infectious Diseases.

What should be done if the septic joint does not get better after the initial surgery?

Occasionally, the patient does not continue to improve despite appropriate surgical and antibiotic treatment. These recalcitrant infections may require two or more surgical irrigation and debridement procedures before significant improvement is made. An MRI scan can be helpful to rule out previously undetected soft-tissue abscess or bony infection in the vicinity of the joint. Either of these should be incised and debrided if detected.

References

1. Massey PA, Clark MD, Walt JS, Feibel BM, Robichaux-Edwards LR, Barton RS. Optimal synovial fluid leukocyte count cutoff for diagnosing native joint septic arthritis after antibiotics: a receiver operating characteristic analysis of accuracy. J Am Acad Orthop Surg. 2021;29(23):e1246–53. https://doi.org/10.5435/JAAOS-D-20-01152.
2. Elsissy JG, Liu JN, Wilton PJ, Nwachuku I, Gowd AK, Amin NH. Bacterial septic arthritis of the adult native knee joint: a review. JBJS Rev. 2020;8(1):e0059. https://doi.org/10.2106/JBJS.RVW.19.00059.
3. Hunter JG, Gross JM, Dahl JD, Amsdell SL, Gorczyca JT. Risk factors for failure of a single surgical debridement in adults with acute septic arthritis. J Bone Joint Surg Am. 2015;97(7):558–64. https://doi.org/10.2106/JBJS.N.00593.

Open Joint Injuries

10

A patient sustains a stab wound near the knee with a dirty knife (Fig. 10.1). The patient has good perfusion and no distal neurologic impairment. Bleeding is controlled by pressure and stops after a few minutes. Does the patient need a tetanus booster?

Tetanus boosters are given every 10 years, but should be given at 5 years for wounds that are "dirty" in the judgment of the treating physician. Given that this was a dirty knife, the patient should receive a tetanus booster if his last booster was more than 5 years ago.

What is the appropriate treatment for penetrating wounds that enter the knee joint?

Penetrating wounds that enter a joint should be treated with irrigation and debridement to minimize the risk of an infection inside the joint [1]. In some cases, the patient may have sustained additional injuries inside the knee that would benefit from surgery, but most of those injuries do not need to be treated urgently. Open joint injury should be treated with urgent irrigation and debridement.

What should be done to evaluate the extent of the injury?

Plain radiographs of the knee should be obtained in order to determine if any metallic particles from the knife blade are in the wound, to examine the bone for any evidence of fracture or injury,

© The Author(s), under exclusive license to Springer Nature
Switzerland AG 2024
J. T. Gorczyca, *Orthopaedic Emergencies*,
https://doi.org/10.1007/978-3-031-62011-9_10

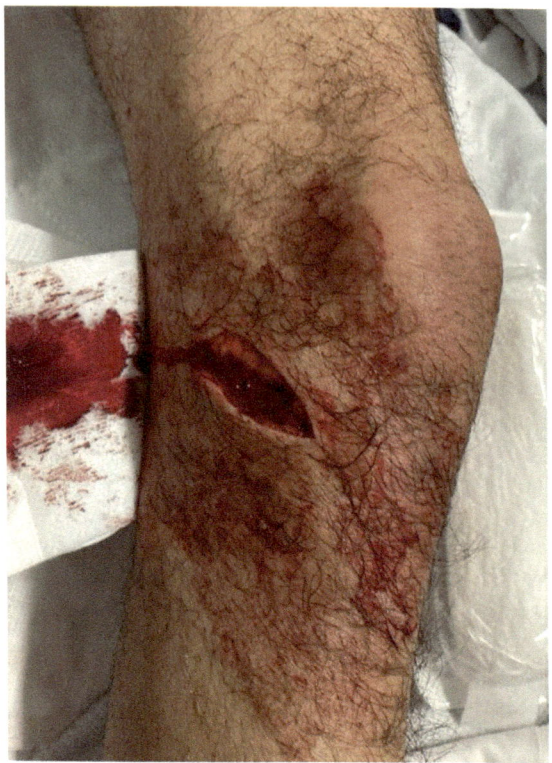

Fig. 10.1 Clinical photo of wound in region of knee. It is unclear whether or not this wound extends into the knee joint, which, if present, would place this patient at risk for septic knee. Thus, further information is needed (photograph courtesy of Brett Salazar, MD)

and to determine if there is any air in the joint, which would indicate that the knife penetrated the knee joint and that surgical irrigation and debridement of the joint should be performed (Fig. 10.2). A CT scan may also demonstrate air in the joint that would indicate the need for surgical debridement and irrigation of the joint.

Additionally, a thorough neurovascular examination should be performed to determine if there is any neurologic or vascular

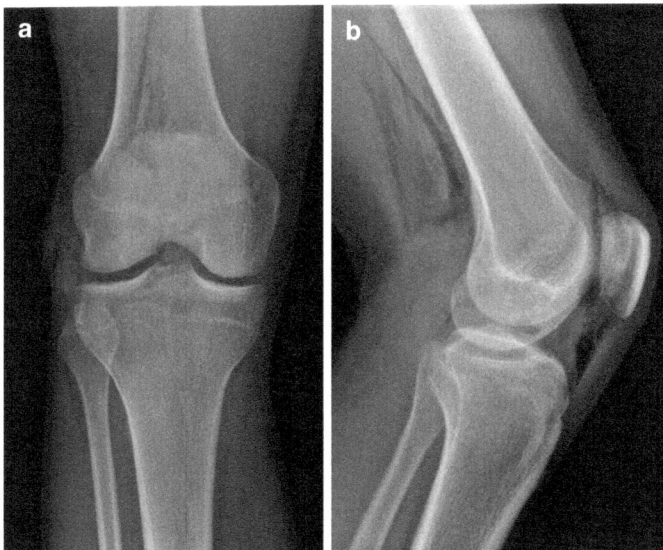

Fig. 10.2 Anteroposterior (**a**) and lateral (**b**) radiographs demonstrate air in the knee joint, which in this case was caused by a traumatic arthrotomy and warrants debridement. Other causes for air in a joint are gas-producing infection as well as recent surgery in the knee joint (radiographs courtesy of Brett Salazar, MD)

injury. Abnormal vascular findings on examination, such as delayed (>3 s) capillary refill or decreased pulses, warrant further investigation with Doppler ultrasound, arteriogram, and/or computed tomographic (CT) angiography.

If the X-rays of the knee are negative, what should be done to assure that the knee joint has not been violated before considering suturing the wound closed?

With a penetrating wound like this, the leg/thigh should be prepped and the knee joint should be injected (through a non-traumatized region) with sterile saline or Lactated Ringer's solution (Fig. 10.3). If after injection of at least 180 cc fluid, there is fluid that drains from inside the knee joint and out through the traumatic wound, the test is positive and indicates that the wound communicates with the joint and intra-articular contamination

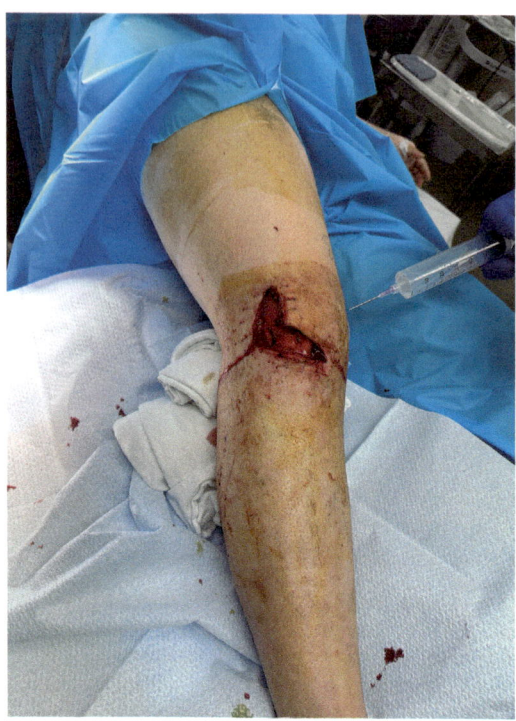

Fig. 10.3 Needle injection of at least 180 cc of sterile fluid into the knee joint provides helpful information. If at least 180 cc of fluid is injected into the knee joint and none leaks out through the traumatic wound, then the study is negative and indicates that a traumatic arthrotomy has occurred. With a positive test, on the other hand, fluid will leak out through the traumatic wound, indicating a traumatic arthrotomy with violation of the knee joint capsule. For a positive test, surgery is indicated to debride and irrigate the knee joint. Irrigation and debridement can be performed arthroscopically or more commonly by open surgical technique

has occurred. In that case, the joint should be irrigated and debrided [2].

What is done at the time of surgery for a traumatic arthrotomy?

If the wound is indeed a traumatic arthrotomy, urgent irrigation and debridement are performed in the OR when the patient is stable enough to tolerate the procedure [1]. An incision is made into the knee joint and the traumatic wound and knee joint are debrided of devitalized tissue and copiously irrigated. Based on the severity of the contamination, the amount of bleeding intraoperatively, and the surgeon's judgment, a decision may be made to place a drain in the joint to remove any fluid postoperatively for a few days. Prophylactic intravenous antibiotics should be administered for a day or two, generally a first generation cephalosporin for smaller and cleaner wound, with gram negative bacterial coverage (e.g., Gentamicin) for larger wounds and anaerobic coverage (e.g., IV Penicillin or clindamycin) for dirty barnyard wounds or wounds with fecal contamination.

Thus, inserting needles into the joint can be helpful diagnostically: For a potential infected knee, a needle is inserted into the wound and the fluid is aspirated and sent for analysis and culture to determine if surgery is indicated. For a potential traumatic arthrotomy, a needle is inserted into the joint and 200 cc of sterile saline is injected to see if a traumatic arthrotomy exists, which is at risk for becoming an infected joint and would indicate that surgery should be performed in order to prevent infection.

References

1. Brubacher JW, Grote CW, Tilley MB. Traumatic arthrotomy. J Am Acad Orthop Surg. 2020;28(3):102–11. https://doi.org/10.5435/JAAOS-D-19-00153.
2. Keese GR, Boody AR, Wongworawat MD, Jobe CM. The accuracy of the saline load test in the diagnosis of traumatic knee arthrotomies. J Orthop Trauma. 2007;21(7):442–3. https://doi.org/10.1097/BOT.0b013-e31812e5186.

Water Wounds

11

A person is walking in muddy water and sustains an irregular, jagged wound to his leg extending to muscle (Fig. 11.1). There is not much bleeding. What are your concerns?

Wounds that are contaminated by open bodies of water are at risk of severe infections. Many lakes and streams, despite appear-

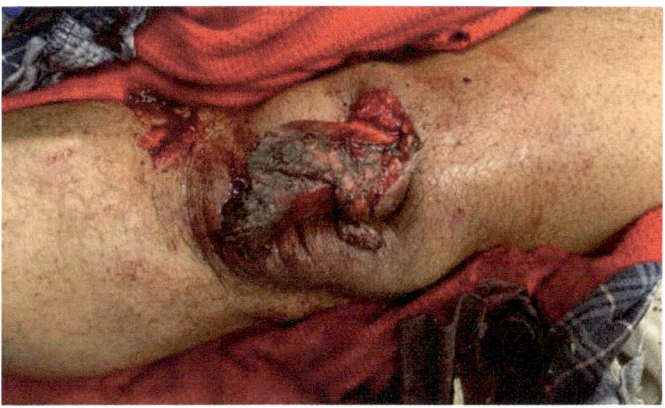

Fig. 11.1 Wound that occurred when the patient was working in muddy water. This wound is at higher risk for infection and should be treated with antibiotics, debrided, irrigated, and left open initially. Delayed primary closure in 2–3 days if the wound appears healthy, or secondary closure by allowing the wound to gradually heal and close over time, are better options for preventing infection (photograph courtesy of Brett Salazar, MD)

J. T. Gorczyca, *Orthopaedic Emergencies*, https://doi.org/10.1007/978-3-031-62011-9_11

ing clean and being open for swimming, harbor bacteria that can aggressively spread in a wound and may require complex antibiotics.

A dirty wound should be treated with a tetanus booster (if not received in the past five years) or tetanus vaccine if the patient has not been vaccinated in the past.

Debridement of devitalized tissue and not closing the wound until the tissue is clean and healthy (i.e. delayed primary wound closure) is the safe way to prevent infection of these wounds [1]. Antibiotics should be provided to treat for gram-positive cocci and gram-negative bacilli.

Many bodies of muddy or cloudy water have fecal contamination, decomposing vegetative material, and complex bacteria and fungi that can infect wounds. Even clean appearing water in lakes or rivers is not sterile and can harbor bacteria that cause severe life-threatening infections. When treating open wounds, it is essential to investigate for history or signs of wound contamination by mud or water, as this could have drastic consequences for the treatment and outcome of the wound.

Figure 11.2 depicts a patient whose arm was repeatedly cut underwater by a rotating boat propeller. What problems do you foresee?

This is a devastating injury with devitalization of a large part of the arm and severe contamination. Despite broad spectrum antibiotic treatment and aggressive irrigation and debridement of devitalized tissue, this patient died from overwhelming sepsis the day after injury.

Fig. 11.2 Open water wound caused by boat propeller with severe tissue destruction and contamination. Despite aggressive surgical debridement and antibiotics, this person died from overwhelming sepsis the day after injury

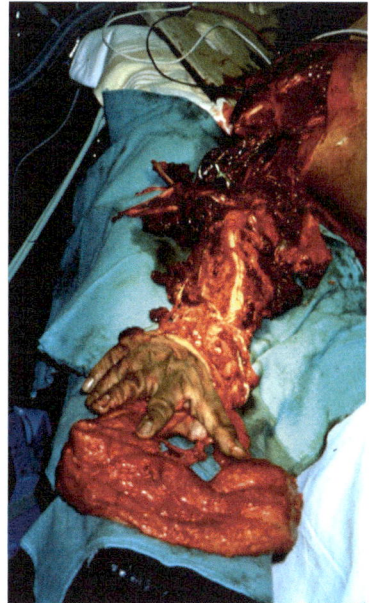

Reference

1. Brophy RH, Bernholt DL. Aquatic orthopaedic injuries. J Am Acad Orthop Surg. 2019;27(6):191–9. https://doi.org/10.5435/JAAOS-D-16-00702.

Displaced Femoral Neck Fractures

A healthy 42-year old woman sustains a hip injury when her motorcycle collides with a utility pole. X-rays are shown in Fig. 12.1. What is the injury, and what is the best treatment?

She has a displaced left femoral neck fracture. After thorough evaluation for associated injuries and stabilization, she should have reduction and operative stabilization of the fracture performed.

This patient has a displaced femoral neck fracture. This fracture should be urgently reduced and stabilized with internal fixation in the operating room [1] (Fig. 12.2).

What complications are more common with this injury compared to other hip fractures?

The location of this fracture at the femoral neck, and the fact that it is displaced, jeopardize the blood supply to the femoral head and place the patient at risk for avascular necrosis as well as nonunion. The blood supply to the femoral head passes through a ring around the base of the femoral neck which sends a series of capsular vessels that pass along the femoral neck toward the femoral head, then penetrate the capsule of the hip joint and enter the femoral neck and head [2]. These vessels may be torn, compressed, clotted, twisted or kinked by the displacement of the fracture at the femoral neck. It is believed that early anatomic reduction of the fracture by closed or direct open means will restore the anatomy of the femoral neck and in some cases, restore perfusion of the femoral head before necrosis of the bone (avascular necrosis) occurs.

© The Author(s), under exclusive license to Springer Nature Switzerland AG 2024
J. T. Gorczyca, *Orthopaedic Emergencies*,
https://doi.org/10.1007/978-3-031-62011-9_12

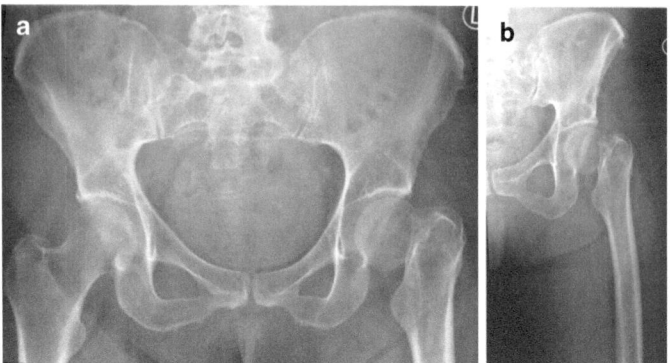

Fig. 12.1 AP pelvis radiograph (**a**) and AP left hip radiograph (**b**) demonstrate displaced left femoral neck fracture

Fig. 12.2 Intraoperative fluoroscopic views demonstrate reduction of the fracture and stabilization with three parallel screws

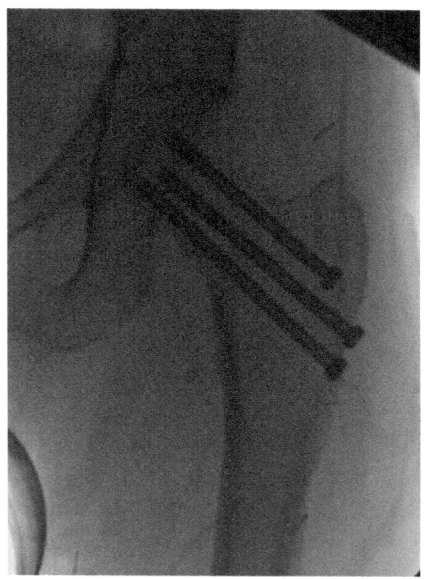

Of note, the artery of the ligamentum teres provides perfusion to the developing femoral head in children, but this artery provides minimal if any perfusion to the femoral head in adults.

Why is necrosis of the femoral head a problem?

Bone is alive and is continually remodeling. Additionally, bone responds to the forces placed applied to it by producing more bone—but it requires blood supply in order to remodel and produce more bone. Additionally, bone sustains microscopic fractures through normal activity; with increasing levels of activity, bone sustains an increased number of microscopic fractures. Healthy, vascularized bone will usually heal these microscopic fractures. Bone that is avascular, however, lacks the ability to heal the microscopic fractures, and with time, the unhealed microscopic fractures will connect with each other and create a macroscopic fracture, which can cause significant pain. This pain can be felt in the hip but is commonly experienced as thigh or knee pain as well (i.e., referred pain).

What can be done to detect avascular necrosis early after a femoral neck fracture?

It is important to understand that patients with femoral neck fractures are at risk of developing avascular necrosis in the months to years following the injury and treatment. Often, early in the progression of avascular necrosis of the femoral head, the patient will have severe pain despite not yet having any sign of avascular necrosis on plain X-rays. In these cases, MRI can be helpful in detecting the AVN before it progresses further (Fig. 12.3a, b). If patients have new onset hip, knee or thigh pain after femoral neck fracture, avascular necrosis of the femoral head should be in the differential diagnosis and radiographs and MRI of the hip should be obtained.

What happens as avascular necrosis progresses?

When the macroscopic fracture in the femoral head does not heal, the pain persists, and inflammation occurs in the area of the fracture which has maintained vascularity. The inflammation will result in resorption of bone and radiographic radiolucency below the articular surface. Eventually, the unsupported bone at the articular surface of the superior femoral head will collapse (Fig. 12.3c, d). Although the cartilage over the femoral head remains healthy (it receives its nutrients and oxygen by diffusion through the joint fluid), when the bone beneath it collapses, the cartilage assumes an irregular contour which will result in irregu-

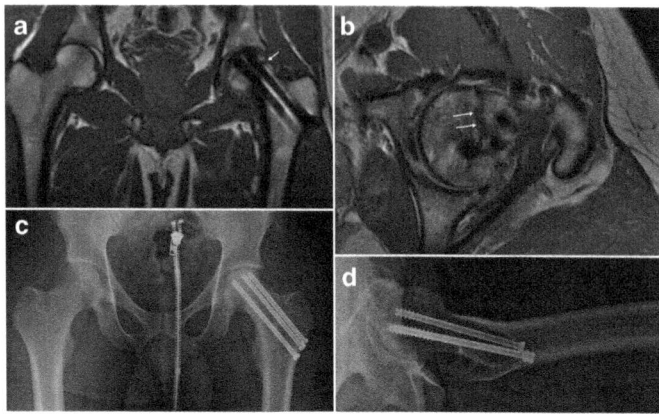

Fig. 12.3 Representative coronal plane (**a**) and axial (**b**) images through femoral head in patient with sudden onset of atraumatic pain in hip 6 months after fracture fixation. Artifact from screws is apparent, and arrows depict the interval between the viable and necrotic bone (AVN) in the femoral head. Three months later, AP pelvis (**c**) and cross table lateral hip (**d**) radiographs show healed femoral neck fracture with relative sclerosis of femoral head. White arrow on AP view demonstrates small step at articular surface consistent with subchondral collapse, while the cross table lateral demonstrates irregular radiographic density at the femoral head without articular incongruity on this view

lar wear of the articular cartilage and eventually osteoarthritis. Often, the pain of the avascular necrosis and fracture is so severe that patients will opt for hip arthroplasty (or other surgery) before there is significant arthritis present on the radiographs.

Why not just treat this fracture with hip replacement, as most patients do very well after this procedure?

Hip arthroplasty is often performed to treat painful osteoarthritis of the hip and is an elective procedure that is associated with a significant improvement in quality of life. After hip arthroplasty, patients who have had pain with normal activity for years, and who had been forced to gradually decrease their activity level and sacrifice doing activities they enjoyed due to the discomfort, are once again able to walk, bicycle, dance, and resume social activities without pain.

Total hip arthroplasty is the standard treatment for older (>60–70 years) patients with displaced femoral neck fractures. Its success in these patients is similar to the success of hip arthroplasty for patients with chronic arthritis. Unfortunately, hip arthroplasty is associated with an infection risk of approximately 1% (which may require one or more operative procedures and the infection may never resolve), a 3% risk of dislocation (which requires anesthesia and closed or open reduction), and a 3% risk of significant thromboembolism despite prophylaxis. The other major risk of hip arthroplasty is aseptic (non-infected) loosening, which with time becomes progressively more painful and eventually warrants revision surgery. As patients get older, they become less active and are less likely to experience aseptic loosening of the hip arthroplasty. In younger, more active patients, the average longevity of hip arthroplasty is 15–25 years [3]. Thus, arthroplasty in this 42-years patient is likely to require a revision procedure before the patient reaches the age of 60, and the longevity of the revision procedure is lower, while the risk of complications is higher. Thus, in younger patients with displaced femoral neck fractures, if the femoral head and the hip joint can be preserved by performing internal fixation, then that would be the best long-term option for the patient.

References

1. Roberts KC, Brox WT, Jevsevar DS, Sevarino K. Management of hip fractures in the elderly. J Am Acad Orthop Surg. 2015;23(2):131–7. https://doi.org/10.5435/JAAOS-D-14-00432.
2. Large TM, Adams MR, Loeffler BJ, Gardner MJ. Posttraumatic avascular necrosis after proximal femur, proximal humerus, talar neck, and scaphoid fractures. J Am Acad Orthop Surg. 2019;27(21):794–805. https://doi.org/10.5435/JAAOS-D-18-00225.
3. Evans JT, Evans JP, Walker RW, Blom AW, Whitehouse MR, Sayers A. How long does a hip replacement last? A systematic review and meta-analysis of case series and national registry reports with more than 15 years of follow-up. Lancet. 2019;393(10172):647–54. https://doi.org/10.1016/S0140-6736(18)31665-9. Epub 2019 Feb 14. PMID: 30782340; PMCID: PMC6376618.

Displaced Talar Neck Fractures

13

A 24-year old laborer sustains a foot injury when he slips while carrying shingles up a ladder and falls down the ladder. A lateral X-ray is shown in Fig. 13.1a. What is the injury, and what is the best treatment?

This patient has a displaced talar neck fracture. This fracture should be urgently reduced (Fig. 13.1b). At some point after reduction, it should be stabilized with internal fixation in the operating room [1].

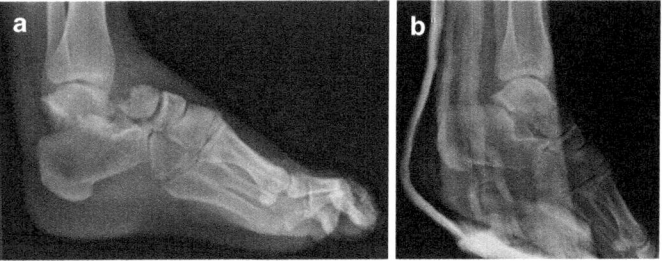

Fig. 13.1 (**a**) Lateral radiograph of the foot and ankle demonstrates a displaced fracture at the talar neck with displacement (dislocation) at the subtalar joint between the posterior talus and calcaneus. (**b**) Lateral radiograph of the foot and ankle after reduction of the fracture and dislocation, with the ankle splinted in plantar flexion to help maintain the reduction

Why is urgent reduction so important?

This fracture is displaced and the posterior subtalar joint (i.e., the joint between the talus and the calcaneus inferior to it) is displaced. Thus, this is a fracture-dislocation. Like many dislocations, the pressure on the skin, neurovascular structures, and cartilage can result in necrosis or irreversible injury if the displacement is not quickly corrected by reduction. Additionally, the blood supply to the body of the talus is often injured or compressed with these displaced fractures, and early reduction of the fracture-dislocation can realign the vessels and improve perfusion of the body of the talus, thereby preventing avascular necrosis [2].

What anatomic features of the talus make it susceptible to avascular necrosis with displaced talar neck fractures?

The talus is located in the middle of the foot and ankle, and articulates with four other bones. Thus, a large percentage (70%) of its surface area is articular cartilage, which generally does not allow for passage of blood vessels to the underlying bone. Also, there are no muscles or tendons that attach to the talus—muscle or tendon attachments are generally good locations through or near which blood vessels can enter a bone. And, the position of the body of the talus within the ankle requires the blood to pass from distally to proximally to reach the body of the talus. There are several other places in the body (femoral head, humeral head, and scaphoid in the wrist) where this retrograde flow places the bone at higher risk for avascular necrosis if a fracture or dislocation occurs and the perfusion is compromised.

What type of injury causes a displaced talar neck fracture?

Talar neck fractures are often caused by hyperdorsiflexion injuries, in which the forced dorsiflexion is so extreme that the anterior aspect of the tibia stops motion of the talar neck, while the continued force causes a fracture as the anterior talus and forefoot continue to displace (Fig. 13.2). As the fracture displaces, there will be displacement of the posterior talus at the subtalar joint. When the displaced forefoot recoils after the traumatic force ceases, the anterior talus will resume its normal location but may

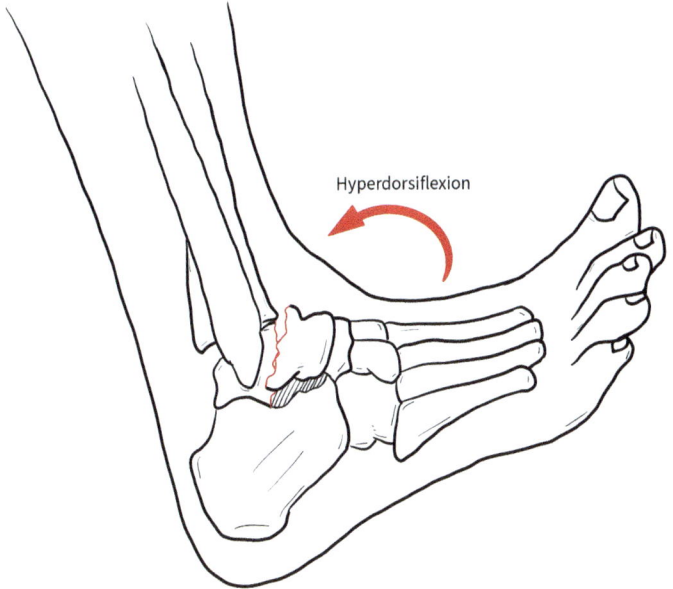

Fig. 13.2 Illustration of mechanism of ankle hyperdorsiflexion and talar neck fracture. (Drawing courtesy of Louis C. Okafor, MD)

force the posterior talus (body) more posteriorly and cause an ankle (tibiotalar) subluxation or dislocation. Of historical interest, displaced talar neck fractures were described in WW II Royal Air Force pilots who sustained hyperdorsiflexion injuries in plane crashes when their foot was forced into dorsiflexion by the rudder bar. The term "aviator's astragalus" was coined for displaced talar neck fractures [3].

What is the surgical treatment for displaced talar neck fractures?

Displaced talar neck fractures should be urgently reduced, and then stabilized anatomically with screws and/or plates. The quality of reduction is critical as any displacement at the fracture will by necessity result in mal-reduction of the posterior portion of the

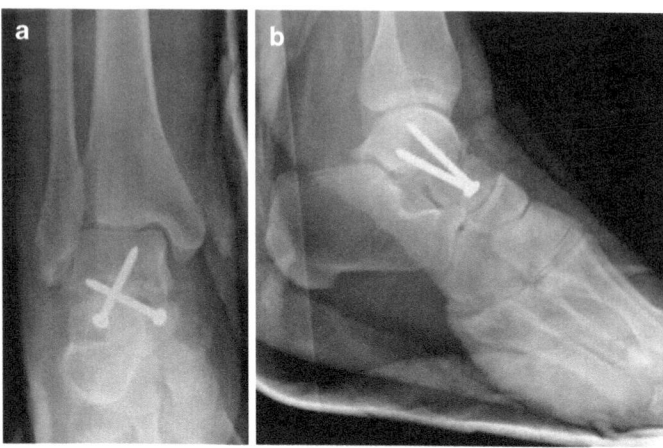

Fig. 13.3 Anteroposterior (**a**) and lateral (**b**) radiographs after open reduction and internal fixation of the displaced talar neck fracture performed through two limited incisions

subtalar joint. Generally, two incisions, one medially and one laterally, are made to view the fracture, and implants are placed through each of the incisions to stabilize the fracture (Fig. 13.3). It is not uncommon in orthopedic surgery to fix a fracture through two incisions, each of which can be performed with limited dissection to preserve the viability of the bone, while allowing visualization of the fracture from two vantage points and allowing improved ability to "fine-tune" the fracture reduction.

The fracture is reduced urgently and stabilized. How will we know if the talar body is experiencing avascular necrosis?

After being treated for displaced talar neck fractures, patients are prohibited from bearing weight for 2–3 months until the fracture heals. During a period of prolonged non-weight bearing or decreased activity, live bone will lose some of its density ("disuse osteopenia"). Thus, at 6–8 weeks after injury, there should be

Fig. 13.4 Mortise view of ankle taken 6 weeks after talar neck fracture. Arrows point to "Hawkins' sign" of subchondral radiolucency in the talar dome due to disuse osteopenia from restricted weight bearing on that foot after the fracture. This is generally a favorable sign as it indicates that avascular necrosis is not present at that location in this patient

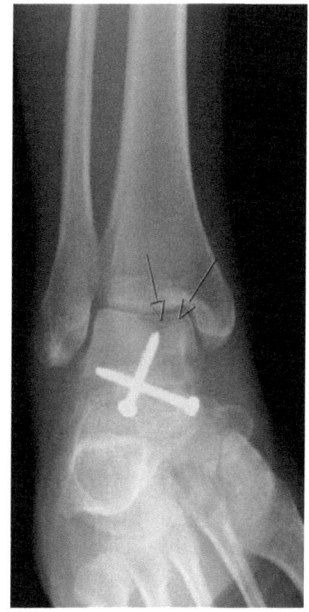

radiographic evidence of disuse osteopenia on X-ray. This finding is best seen as subchondral radiolucency on the ankle mortise X-ray (Fig. 13.4). The lack of density is a good sign, as it indicates that the bone is viable and is responding normally to the decreased forces placed on it. The bone density and strength will gradually return to normal after the fracture heals when the patient resumes weight bearing and normal activity (Fig. 13.5). Sometimes, if the patient has impaired perfusion to the bone, the subchondral radiolucency may not occur for many months after the fracture. If the subchondral radiolucency from revascularization never appears, then the patient has avascular necrosis and is more likely to experience arthritis and pain as a consequence.

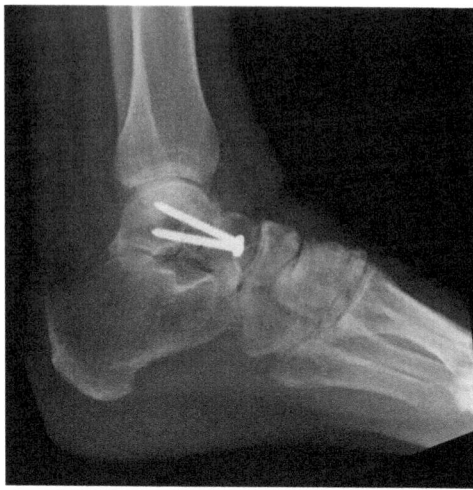

Fig. 13.5 3-month postoperative lateral ankle radiographs demonstrate good maintenance of alignment and healing of fracture

References

1. Lee C, Brodke D, Perdue PW Jr, Patel T. Talus fractures: evaluation and treatment. J Am Acad Orthop Surg. 2020;28(20):e878–87. https://doi.org/10.5435/JAAOS-D-20-00116.
2. Large TM, Adams MR, Loeffler BJ, Gardner MJ. Posttraumatic avascular necrosis after proximal femur, proximal humerus, talar neck, and scaphoid fractures. J Am Acad Orthop Surg. 2019;27(21):794–805. https://doi.org/10.5435/JAAOS-D-18-00225.
3. Coltart WD. Aviator's astragalus. J Bone Joint Surg Br. 1952;34(4):545–66. https://doi.org/10.1302/0301-620X.34B4.545.

Slipped Capital Femoral Epiphysis

14

A 7-year old girl complains of gradual onset of knee pain. There was no injury. She is unable to walk. What should be done?

Any time a child is unable to walk, they should be evaluated by an orthopaedist. Joint infection, fracture, growth plate abnormality, and tumor need to be considered and ruled out.

Problems occurring in the hip in children will cause pain in the hip as well as pain that is referred to the thigh or knee. Thus, children who cannot walk and have knee or thigh pain should have radiographs of the hip and femur as well as of the knee.

The patient was afebrile and had normal laboratory studies (CBC, CRP, and ESR). Hip radiographs were obtained (Fig. 14.1). What should be done now?

The radiograph has the subtle finding of minimal angulation through the right proximal femoral physis (growth plate), also known as slipped capital femoral epiphysis (SCFE). The patient should be admitted to a hospital, placed on bed rest, and prepared for surgery to stabilize SCFE [1].

Unfortunately, the radiographic findings were not appreciated and the patient was sent home with crutches. She returned to the hospital the next day with more pain and the following radiographs were obtained (Fig. 14.2). What do you see now?

The epiphysis has slipped (displaced) even farther now. The angulation on the lateral radiograph of the hip is fairly obvious.

© The Author(s), under exclusive license to Springer Nature Switzerland AG 2024
J. T. Gorczyca, *Orthopaedic Emergencies*,
https://doi.org/10.1007/978-3-031-62011-9_14

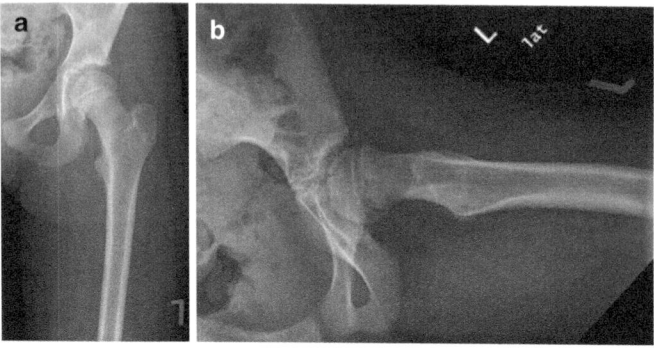

Fig. 14.1 (**a**) Anteroposterior (AP) hip radiograph in a 7-year-old child with left hip pain and inability to walk show no significant abnormality. (**b**) Frog leg lateral radiograph of the hip shows slight posterior displacement (slip) through the physis (growth plate)

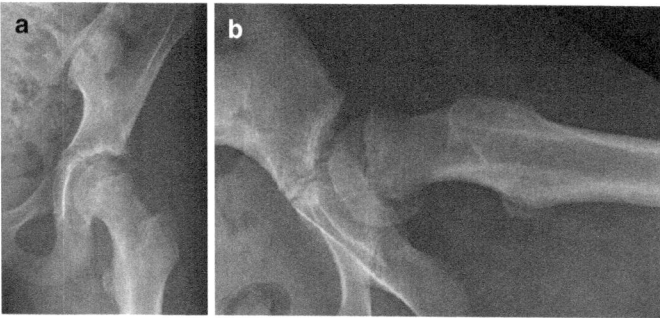

Fig. 14.2 (**a**) AP hip radiograph the next day shows minimal change. (**b**) Frog leg lateral hip radiograph, however, shows significant posterior displacement of femoral head (epiphysis) at the physis (slipped capital femoral epiphysis)

This would have been prevented if the correct diagnosis had been made initially and the patient was protected by restricting hip motion.

What should be done to treat the hip problem?

The SCFE should be surgically stabilized to prevent further displacement and to allow healing. This is performed in the operating room using a screw placed percutaneously (i.e., through very small incisions) with fluoroscopic guidance [1, 2]. The patient is restricted from bearing weight until there is clinical and radiographic evidence of healing.

What are the complications of SCFE?

The complication of SCFE that is most concerning is avascular necrosis, which occurs more commonly when the physis has displaced or when the patient is unable to walk, both of which became risk factors in this patient. The exact pathophysiology on the avascular necrosis is unclear but is related to alteration in the blood flow to the femoral head.

Why is avascular necrosis of the femoral head a problem?

As explained in the chapter on joint dislocations and on displaced femoral neck fractures, bone is alive and is constantly remodeling and repairing microscopic fractures which occur in the course of normal activity. Avascular bone lacks the capacity to heal these microfractures. Thus, the microfractures eventually connect to become macrofractures, which cause pain and trigger an inflammatory response that resorbs bone. When bone beneath the articular surface is resorbed, the joint surface collapses and becomes irregular (Fig. 14.3), eventually leading to joint destruction and osteoarthritis. The treatment options for avascular necro-

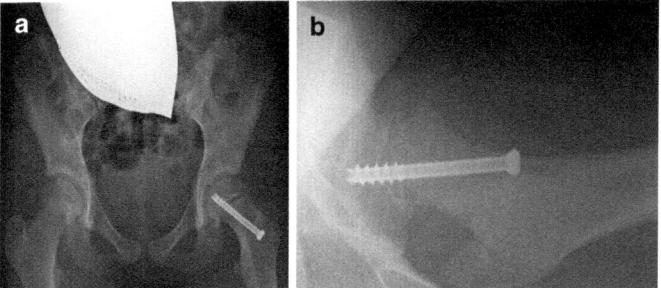

Fig. 14.3 AP pelvis (**a**) and frog leg lateral (**b**) pelvis radiographs after operative stabilization of the slipped capital femoral epiphysis. Reduction of the displacement was not performed as it can cause further damage to the blood supply and a higher rate of avascular necrosis of the femoral head

sis are limited. The best treatment is prevention by early detection and treatment.

What causes SCFE?

SCFE occurs because the cartilage is weaker than usual. Several endocrine diseases are associated with SCFE, including hypothyroidism, growth hormone deficiency, and pituitary tumors. Additionally, chronic diseases, renal osteodystrophy, puberty, and obesity are associated with SCFE [3].

Thus, thorough endocrinological evaluation to rule out underlying disease is essential in the ongoing treatment of these patients.

Is there anything else to consider in the treatment of these patients?

The same factors that caused SCFE in the one hip will place the patient at risk for contralateral involvement. About 20% of patients initially present with bilateral SCFE, and another 20–40% will progress to contralateral involvement in the future. Thus, serious consideration of prophylactic fixation of the uninvolved hip should be made. This can generally be delayed until the patient is able to bear weight on the involved side. If the patient begins to experience pain in the contralateral hip (or thigh or knee), then this should be interpreted as impending SCFE and the hip should be stabilized at that time to prevent displacement of the contralateral SCFE (Fig. 14.4).

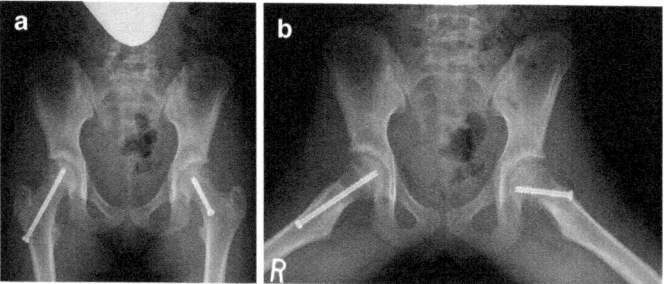

Fig. 14.4 The patient began having right hip pain 3 weeks after the left hip surgery. Radiographs showed no change in alignment. A decision was made to perform stabilization of the right hip, as demonstrated by the postoperative AP pelvis (**a**) and frog leg lateral pelvis (**b**) radiographs

In summary, SCFE often occurs in overweight adolescents, but it can occur in slender and younger children as well. The patient may complain of pain in the hip, thigh or knee. X-rays, including frog leg lateral radiographs of the hip, are essential to making the diagnosis. Risk factors for poor results are displaced SCFE and inability to walk. Surgical stabilization is necessary, and most patients should have surgery on both sides, even if asymptomatic on the contralateral side. Every patient with SCFE should undergo a thorough Endocrine evaluation to detect and treat any previously diagnosed endocrine disorders. SCFE commonly occurs in adolescent patients, but can occur in younger patients like the 7-year old girl presented in this chapter.

References

1. Aronsson DD, Loder RT, Breur GJ, Weinstein SL. Slipped capital femoral epiphysis: current concepts. J Am Acad Orthop Surg. 2006;14(12):666–79. https://doi.org/10.5435/00124635-200611000-00010.
2. Kuzyk PR, Kim YJ, Millis MB. Surgical management of healed slipped capital femoral epiphysis. J Am Acad Orthop Surg. 2011;19(11):667–77. https://doi.org/10.5435/00124635-201111000-00003.
3. Witbreuk M, van Kemenade FJ, van der Sluijs JA, Jansma EP, Rotteveel J, van Royen BJ. Slipped capital femoral epiphysis and its association with endocrine, metabolic and chronic diseases: a systematic review of the literature. J Child Orthop. 2013;7(3):213–23. https://doi.org/10.1007/s11832-013-0493-8. Epub 2013 Mar 30. PMID: 24432080; PMCID: PMC3672463.

Compartment Syndrome

15

A 36-year-old pedestrian is struck by a car and sustains a closed tibia fracture. She has no sign of neurovascular injury (Fig. 15.1). Her tibia was reduced and placed in a circumferential long leg cast. Three hours later, the pain in her leg is severe and is not improving with narcotic medication. What should be done next?

This patient is at risk for compartment syndrome from swelling of the muscle and from bleeding within the compartments of the leg. The circumferential, rigid cast is also a factor as it lacks the capacity to expand. The cast should be bivalved (completely cut with a cast saw on two sides) and the padding released down to the skin on both sides to allow the leg to expand and the pain to subside. The patient should be re-examined in 5–10 min to see if the pain has improved and if the patient has normal neurologic and vascular function in the extremity.

What is compartment syndrome?

Compartment syndrome is a clinical situation in which pressure within an anatomic area, such as within muscle compartments, is so high that it blocks perfusion of the muscle through the microvasculature—usually the perfusion is blocked at the capillaries, where the pressure is lowest [1, 2].

The compromised perfusion of tissue causes ischemia, pain, and more swelling, which will eventually progress to irreversible necrosis of the tissue in the compartments if the process is not

© The Author(s), under exclusive license to Springer Nature
Switzerland AG 2024
J. T. Gorczyca, *Orthopaedic Emergencies*,
https://doi.org/10.1007/978-3-031-62011-9_15

Fig. 15.1 High-energy tibial plateau fracture that can be associated with compartment syndrome. This injury presents a diagnostic obstacle because the pain from the fracture can be difficult to distinguish from the pain caused by compartment syndrome

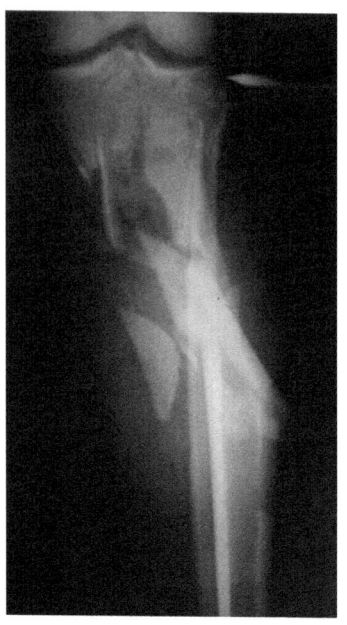

interrupted. It is up to the medical team to recognize the risk of compartment syndrome, to monitor the patient, to identify compartment syndrome as soon as it occurs, and to quickly treat the compartment syndrome surgically to prevent muscle necrosis.

What injuries are most commonly associated with compartment syndrome?

While any injury to an extremity can cause compartment syndrome, fractures of the tibia and fractures of the radius are the most common. Crushing injuries which create significant damage to an extremity, even without a fracture, are also associated with significant swelling and compartment syndrome.

What are other risk factors for compartment syndrome?

Open fractures are more commonly associated with compartment syndrome. This is a bit counter-intuitive, as the open fracture may allow some blood to leave the extremity and decrease the compartment pressure. However, the open fracture wound usually does not release pressure in the entire compartment, and the increased trauma that causes the open fracture is likely to cause more injury to the tissues, and thus more swelling, which explains the higher incidence of compartment syndrome in open fractures.

Coagulopathy can increase the risk of bleeding into a compartment, even with low energy trauma and without a fracture [3]. This is a significant concern because many patients, especially older patients, receive treatment with anticoagulants for atrial fibrillation, thromboembolism, prosthetic heart valves, etc. Generally, treatment with anticoagulants does not cause clinical problems. However, in some patients who are being treated with therapeutic or prophylactic anticoagulation, a seemingly minor injury can cause significant hemorrhage into a compartment which can result in compartment syndrome.

Reperfusion of a previously ischemic limb can cause swelling significant enough to create compartment syndrome. This is the reason that many vascular surgeons will perform a prophylactic fasciotomy after revascularizing an ischemic limb. Patients who have had inadequate tissue perfusion due to septic or hypovolemic shock are also at risk for compartment syndrome after they are resuscitated and perfusion to the extremity is restored; this can occur even if there was no traumatic injury to the extremity.

As stated above, a non-expansive cast can create a compartment syndrome that responds to bivalving the cast and releasing the underlying padding. Similarly, a dressing on an extremity that is too tight can cause compartment syndrome, even in an extremity with minimal injury.

What are the symptoms and signs of compartment syndrome?

Patients with compartment syndrome will experience severe pain in the extremity if they are awake and responsive. With time, they may develop sensory loss and loss function of the muscles in that compartment. Physical examination often reveals swelling in the leg, with tightness in the compartments (Fig. 15.2). The muscle will be tender to pressure. Stretching the involved muscle by passively moving the associated joint will cause pain in that muscle.

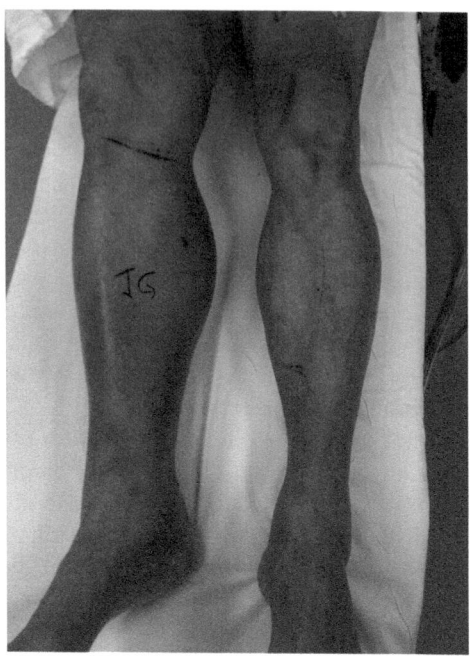

Fig. 15.2 Clinical photograph demonstrates swollen right leg in patient with compartment syndrome. Note the contrast with the size of the other leg due to the swelling

What are some factors that make diagnosis of compartment syndrome difficult?

There are several factors that complicate the evaluation of patients with compartment syndrome. First, the skin may appear completely normal, with normal capillary perfusion. This is often the case because the skin is outside the compartment, so its perfusion is unaffected by the compartment syndrome. Second, the patient will usually have a palpable pulse, as the pressure in the artery is much higher than the pressure in the compartment which it traverses. The arteriolar and capillary pressure is much more likely to be occluded by elevated compartment pressure, thereby resulting in tissue ischemia even when the arterial pulse is palpable. Third, some compartments are deep and may not feel tense, especially in patients with abundant subcutaneous adipose tissue, so the leg may feel soft even in a patient with all the other signs of compartment syndrome. Fourth, the patient may be obtunded or have a nerve injury that makes them less likely to show signs and symptoms of compartment syndrome. Fifth, many patients have significant injuries to the extremity that cloud the diagnosis because they cause swelling, tenderness to pressure, and pain on passive stretch, even though the swelling is not significant enough to cause compartment syndrome. Finally, compartment syndrome can evolve quickly or gradually, and continued monitoring and re-examination will be necessary to detect it as early as possible.

What should be done if the diagnosis of compartment syndrome is unclear?

When it is unclear whether or not the patient has compartment syndrome, measuring the pressure in the involved compartment(s) will provide helpful information [1, 2, 4]. If the difference between the patient's diastolic blood pressure and the compartment pressure (i.e., ΔP) is less than 30 mmHg, then the pressure gradient is likely to be too low to provide adequate tissue perfusion, and tissue necrosis will occur unless the muscle compartment is surgically released by performing fasciotomy.

The intracompartmental pressure can be measured with a hand-held pressure monitor or with an arterial line pressure monitor, either of which can be attached by tubing to a special needle inserted into the compartment in question (Fig. 15.3 Stryker monitor)

If the patient is in a hospital that does not have an orthopedic surgeon that can perform the urgent fasciotomy surgery if necessary, then the patient should be transferred as soon as possible to a trauma center that will be able to provide ongoing evaluation and urgent fasciotomy.

What should be done once a compartment syndrome is diagnosed?

The patient with compartment syndrome should undergo emergent release (i.e., fasciotomy) of any compartment involved. The leg has four compartments, all of which are generally released when a diagnosis of compartment syndrome is established in one or more of those compartments. The arm, and thigh each have two

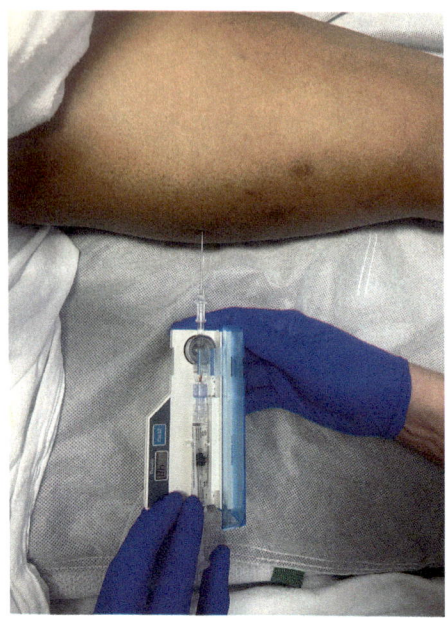

Fig. 15.3 Handheld compartment pressure instrument being used to measure compartment pressures in the thigh (photograph courtesy of Amy Phan, MD)

compartments that may need to be released. The forearm has two compartments, and many surgeons will also release the brachioradialis fascia and perform a carpal tunnel release at the time of forearm fasciotomy. Fasciotomy is performed by making a longitudinal incision first in the skin, and then through the underlying fascia around each muscle group (Fig. 15.4). Each compartment is incised longitudinally to alleviate the pressure on the muscle in the entire compartment. It is tempting to make short incisions, but the fasciotomy incision must be long enough to decompress the entire compartment, so these skin and fascial incisions are usually almost the entire length of the muscle in the compartment(s).

After fasciotomy is performed, what is done with the incisions?

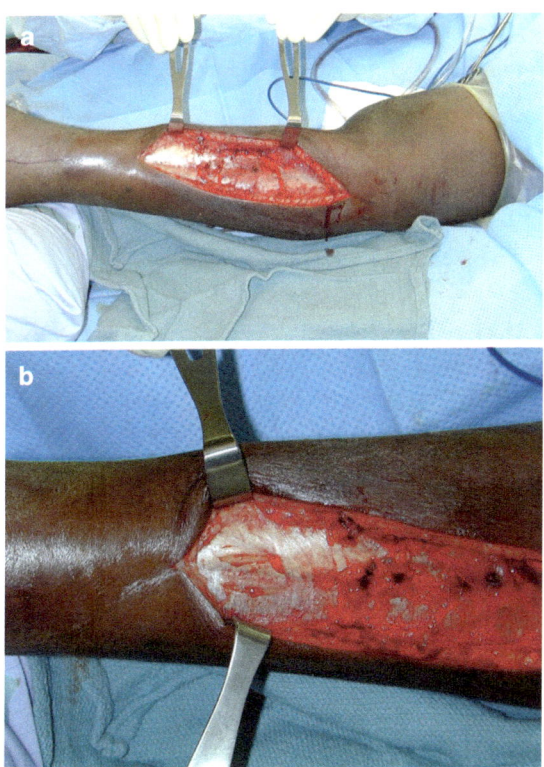

Fig. 15.4 (**a**) Clinical photograph demonstrates incision through lateral skin incision but not yet into the compartments. (**b**) Initial incisions into the lateral and anterior compartments of the leg

Any fractures in the region should be stabilized with internal or external fixation. The fascial and skin incisions are left open until the swelling subsides enough to allow closure, which generally takes 2–5 days. Often, a criss-cross elastic and or vessel loop can be used to gently pull the skin edges toward each other in order to prevent skin retraction and to facilitate wound closure at a later date (Fig. 15.5). A sterile dressing or negative pressure dressing is applied to keep the wound clean. The patient is taken

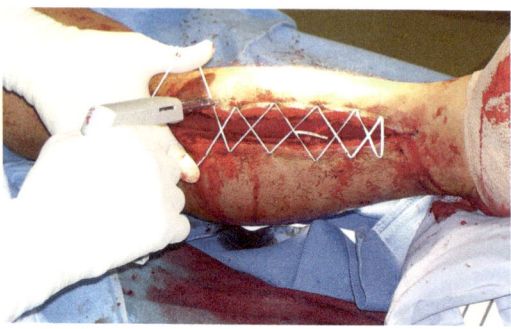

Fig. 15.5 Criss-cross vessel loops or elastic bands can be used to maintain gentle traction on the skin after fasciotomy. This may prevent retraction of the skin and avoid the need for skin grafting

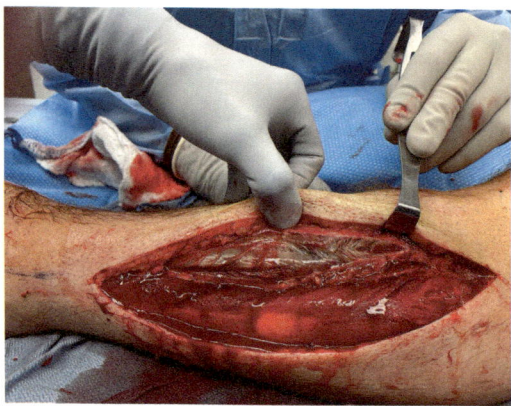

Fig. 15.6 Clinical photograph of leg shows necrotic muscle in patient who had delayed diagnosis and treatment of compartment syndrome

back to the OR in 2–3 days to irrigate the wounds, debride any devitalized tissue (Fig. 15.6), and perform closure of one or both wounds if it can be done without excessive tension on the skin edges. The patient generally returns to the OR every 2–3 days until the wounds can be closed or skin grafting is performed to cover the soft-tissue defect.

References

1. Olson SA, Glasgow RR. Acute compartment syndrome in lower extremity musculoskeletal trauma. J Am Acad Orthop Surg. 2005;13(7):436–44. https://doi.org/10.5435/00124635-200511000-00003.
2. Osborn CPM, Schmidt AH. Management of acute compartment syndrome. J Am Acad Orthop Surg. 2020;28(3):e108–14. https://doi.org/10.5435/JAAOS-D-19-00270.
3. Bauer TW, Resnick L. Coagulopathic complications in orthopaedics. JBJS Case Connect. 2019;9(2):e0266. https://doi.org/10.2106/JBJS.CC.19.00266.
4. Roberts CS, Gorczyca JT, Ring D, Pugh KJ. Diagnosis and treatment of less common compartment syndromes of the upper and lower extremities: current evidence and best practices. Instr Course Lect. 2011;60:43–50.

Index

© The Editor(s) (if applicable) and The Author(s), under exclusive license to Springer Nature Switzerland AG 2024
J. T. Gorczyca, *Orthopaedic Emergencies*,
https://doi.org/10.1007/978-3-031-62011-9